THE SOUL OF MEDICINE

*A Physician's Exploration of Death
and the Question of Being Human*

James I. Raymond, MD

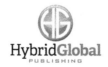

HybridGlobal
PUBLISHING

Published by
Hybrid Global Publishing
301 E 57th Street, 4th fl
New York, NY 10022

Manufactured in the United States of America, or in the United Kingdom when distributed elsewhere.

Raymond, James
   *The Soul of Medicine: A Physician's Exploration of Death
   and the Question of Being Human*
   LCCN: 2018963539
   ISBN: 978-1-948181-27-3
   eBook: 978-1-948181-28-0

Cover design: Joe Potter / joepotter.com
Copyediting: Claudia Volkman
Interior design: Claudia Volkman
Photo credits: Joshua Aaron Photography / joshuaaaronphotography.com

DEDICATION

To Stephanie Hall, James Reinertsen, MD,
and George Khushf, PhD

In 1959 Bertrand Russell wrote several essays focusing on the "expand-ing mental universe." In simplistic terms there are three functional components of this "universe": 1) Thinking, 2) Willing, and 3) Feeling. Ideally, all three components must grow in tandem. [Heretofore most growth and progress has occurred in the area of Thinking. Russell makes the point that only "cultivating cleverness" will be disastrous in the long range and will lead humanity toward its eventual extinction. To be effective, all three components must grow concomitantly.] The three individuals to whom this work is dedicated display all three com-ponents in their proper proportion.

CONTENTS

FOREWORD

SOME YEARS AGO, when we were both on the American Board of Internal Medicine, Dick Leblond and I had a long conversation (aided by a glass or two of an excellent Pinot Noir) exploring the question, "Is there anything that practitioners of the medical arts down through the centuries, and across continents and cultures, have had in common? Do modern science-based doctors do anything similar to what Mesopotamian priests, Roman entrails readers, and Zulu shamans did?"

Dick posited that there has been one constant: all medical practitioners, through all ages, have been expected to answer three questions asked by their patients:

1) What is happening to me?
2) What is going to happen to me?
3) Can you change my future for the better?

As we talked, we realized that the first question is not just about a diagnosis—a "what"—but also about the "why." To address the "what" question, modern doctors must uncover and interpret patterns in signs and symptoms, radiologic images and laboratory reports. But to fully address the question, including "why," doctors have always needed understand the cultural, familial, and religious/spiritual milieu in which their patients are experiencing their illness.

The second question, similarly, we decided is not simply about what we might term a "prognosis." To do a good job with questions such as "Will I ever play hockey again?" "Can I ever have a baby?" and "Will I live long enough to see my grandchild graduate high school?" one must do more than study life-table analyses and case reports in medical journals. Good doctors, for thousands of years, have needed to set their answers into the frame of each patient's hopes, fears, and dreams.

We concluded that there is one profound difference between modern doctors and our predecessors: we are now able to answer the third question—"Can you change my future for the better?"—in the affirmative, confidently, backed by evidence. Our predecessors used herbs, potions, stargazing, entrails reading, mumbo jumbo, and the placebo effect—not much firepower when faced with meningitis, two feet of infarcted bowel, or melanoma. In contrast, we now have effective treatments based on science for well over half of all the named diseases and conditions, and we should be proud of that. It is the glory of modern medicine. But Dick and I also felt that with this new power has come a strong temptation—to be so focused on our newfound ability to change patients' futures for the better that we have lost sight of the importance, and complexity, of the first two questions. And as doctors, we might also have been so enthralled by our scientific prowess that we have forgotten that, with respect to the third question, one of our most important roles has always been to heal, even when we cannot cure.

In essence, we cannot address any of these three questions well if we do not understand what gives meaning to each patient's existence, and to our own. And that requires two things often lacking in modern practice: time and touch. We need enough time to listen to and reflect on our patients' stories, beliefs, and fears, and relate them to our own. And we need to be close enough to those patients to reach out, touch them on the arm, and say, "Tell me more about that," at critical moments in our interactions. Because that's when the magic happens—when we get to the real issues, the heart of the matter.

I often wish that Jim Raymond had been in our conversation. I have no doubt that he would have agreed with Dr. Leblond and me that modern doctors have been so entranced by their ability to answer the third question that they often deal superficially with the first two. And after the experience of working closely with Jim for over a decade, I think he would have stretched our thinking; he would have pointed out that it is difficult to build relationships capable of supporting healing and understand what gives meaning to our patients' existence when we devote so much time and attention in modern professional life to the science and business of medicine: data, evidence, documentation, productivity, and Pay for Performance. As I read Dr. Raymond's powerful story of "The Major" in this book, for example, I could not help reflecting on how unlikely it would be that a modern doctor-in-training would ever take the time for such a profound (and life-changing, for the physician!) series of conversations with a patient.

I think that Jim, with his stunning erudition and gentle manner, would also have pushed Dick Leblond and me a bit on the "doctor-centric" nature of our discussion. It's very clear from his lifetime example as a practicing physician, from the doctor-patient narratives in this astonishingly honest book, and from his deep philosophical exploration of what it is to be human that Jim Raymond believes that the core process involved in being a doctor—building relationships capable of supporting healing—goes both ways. Just as physicians can support the healing of patients, patients can support the healing of physicians. And if we focus solely on the science and business of medicine, driving philosophical and moral reflection out of our daily lives, we physicians will fail to experience the insights, wisdom, and healing that deep relationships with our patients might have brought about. Through his stories, Dr. Raymond brings us right to the heart of what is today termed "patient-centeredness:" we doctors have as much to gain from our patients as they have to gain from us. Perhaps all those who are worried about the apparent epidemic of burnout in our profession would benefit from reading this book, and from reflecting on what we must do within our profession to restore time and touch with our patients, so that we physicians can begin healing ourselves.

Who else might want to read this book? First and most obvious, anyone involved in or contemplating entering the profession of medicine should experience this "unreadable" book. I predict that it will soon become core reading, along with Samuel Shem's House of God, for medical school courses with titles such as "Medicine and the Humanities." But I also believe that the readership of this gem will extend far beyond the medical profession, because, even though Jim Raymond views the question through a doctor's eye, this book speaks profoundly to all of us on the much broader question of what it means to be fully human. Besides, in its own peculiar and disturbing way, "being-towards-death" turns out to be the heart of a damn good story.

One more thought before you start reading: Why did Jim Raymond write this? I believe that Dr. Raymond wrote this book to confront doctors with the following choice: Will my practice of medicine be driven primarily by the rigors of science and the tyranny of business? Or will my practice be guided by the timeless, fundamental role of physicians to build relationships capable of supporting healing, one by one, with our patients?

I also believe that he wrote it to provoke our entire profession to face an even more difficult question, along the lines of Kant's first metaphysical postulate: Does medicine still have a soul? To start understanding the answer, turn the page.

James L. Reinertsen, MD
October 2018
Alta, Wyoming

INTRODUCTION

I FIRST MET Jim Raymond during an interview for a job with Palmetto Health's Center for Bioethics. After Richland Memorial Hospital merged with Baptist Hospital, he became the chief medical and academic officer of Palmetto Health, the largest health system in the Midlands of South Carolina, the organization that was funding the center. He would shepherd the development of quality initiatives for the next couple of decades. Normally, a bioethicist could not expect to find much of a sympathetic ear for the topics associated with my interests. But when I entered his office, books on philosophy and history lined the walls. I thought to myself: *This will be a fun interview! How nice to find such a physician!*

I was wrong about the interview. It was not fun. In fact, it was the worst, most painful interview I ever had. I remember it as a strange form of torture. After I sat down, Dr. Raymond just looked at me. No matter what I said, there was just silence and his attentive stare. All I remember is the silence. It lasted forever. I was just squirming in the seat, trying to find something to say that might get him more engaged. I started over and over from a hundred different directions, but there was no response. It was like having an interview with a corpse—a strange, uncanny kind of corpse that has its eyes open and stares right through you. He could not be moved to speak. So, at least, it seemed at the time.

Somehow I got the job. As I came to know the person, I discovered that he interrogates everything, including himself, in the same troubling, uncomfortable way he interviewed me. I also learned that behind his silence and stare is the most remarkable kind of listening. His silence is strategic, oriented toward just those features of the world that normally lie outside the attention and language of everyday discourse. His silence is the echo of what is unsaid in the world. As he attentively hovers at the awkward, anxious places of life, somehow the normally unsaid aspects of that life emerge and stumble forth into language. In this art of conveying what is yet to be said, both Jim's words and his life are poetic in the sense conveyed by his guide from the grave, Martin Heidegger: through his language a home is constructed where the unsaid things come to dwell. As we think along with these words, we may come to appreciate where our own attention should be directed. Thus, the words of someone on an authentic quest orient us in our own quests and questioning.

In this book, Jim Raymond conveys to us what he sees and hears at those uncomfortable places where most people do not want to linger, look, and listen. In doing this, he explores what the standard languages of science, medicine, and management do not and cannot understand and express. His story takes the form of an autobiographical narrative: how, in his journey, he became disenchanted with a medical science that refuses to reflect upon and acknowledge its own limits. Modern medicine reduced to merely its scientific parts is, as the title of this book indicates, a medicine that has lost its soul. As Jim struggles with his own pain and suffering, mortality, addiction, and all of the other disappointments and failures of life, he also explores the various alternative languages we have for making sense of who we are as humans. He considers the resources of myth, poetry, literature, and philosophy, and finds in each insights that can inform how we are to respond in fitting ways to the brokenness we encounter in our daily lives.

At one level this is an autobiographical work. But it is clearly much more than that. The journey of Dr. Raymond's life and his effort to make sense of it as a quest oriented toward confronting and transcending his own failures, limits, and mortality is simultaneously and in a remarkable way also the journey of contemporary medicine. Admittedly, it is not the outward, well-known, celebrated journey of contemporary medicine. It is not about its heroic successes. Rather, this is the journey of medicine at the hidden places, where physicians wake up, become honest, and frankly face up to all the limits and failures that daily play out in every healthcare setting. Even more, this is the journey of a person, a physician, and a representative of medicine who rediscovers a richer set of resources for discerning what is to be valued in these places where we encounter real people who are compelled to confront their own mortality in the midst of the suffering that attends illness.

What exactly a fitting response requires remains an open question. Through his brutally honest reflections on his own failings, we never get pat answers to standard questions. Instead we glimpse the real questions, the kind we should be asking but often lack the courage to confront. But those who learn to ask in the way Jim Raymond does will find themselves at the place where a fitting human response may arise. This is a deeply ethical work: it brings us to a clearing where the genuine work of ethics can properly take place. Those interested in bioethics can find here a rich inspiration for discovering just those things we need to honestly think forward if what we do is to matter.

There is, surprisingly, a persist hopeful theme that Dr. Raymond clearly articulates in his prologue: "What at first appears 'like the toad, ugly and venomous,' is found at last to wear 'a precious jewel in his head.'" But he should have warned us: this wonderful inversion does not happen automatically. It depends on struggling with those ugly and venomous parts in an authentic way. How fortunate I was to have that terrible interview and be tutored by that painful silence! I can attest to the hope he speaks about. So too for readers of this work: an exciting quest awaits those who are willing to pause and listen for the unsaid things and struggle to read the unreadable book in the right way.

George Khushf, PhD
Professor and Director
Center for Bioethics
University of South Carolina

AUTHOR'S NOTE

"I, TOO, SEEK an unreadable book." So opens the late Robert Nozick's *Philosophical Explanations.*[1] It's unreadable, not because it's poorly written or excessively technical, but because it contains "urgent thoughts to grapple with in agitation and excitement, revelations to be transformed by or to transform, a book incapable of being read straight through, a book, even, to bring reading to a stop."

I mused about the "unreadable" book before I came across Nozick. In fact, one of my personal goals in life has been (and still is) to identify one. I've come very close but have never quite gotten there. That said, I hope I've made this work as "unreadable" as possible.

PROLOGUE

. . . Students waken trembling in their beds
. . . Chilled in the heart by the mailman
With a letter from an aging white haired General
Director of Selection for service in Deathwar
All this black language
Writ by machine!
O hopeless Fathers and Teachers
In Hué do you know the same woe too?
FROM "WICHITA VORTEX SUTRA," ALLEN GINSBERG, 1966

EACH GENERATION HAS a defining event—a watershed separating past innocence from future worldliness—a "before and after" by which time is gauged. Mine was the conflict in Vietnam. As with all wars, it affected society-at-large by gradually resetting its collective unconscious. For its draft-age participants, however, the impact was more sudden and substantial: it "dislocated" lives. (The word *dislocate* seems especially appropriate, even removed from its usual medical context. As the "forceful displacement of something from its normal position," it can be applied as well to a life deflected from its path as to a bone pulled from its socket.) Considering the millions of dislocations it caused, a solitary story is insignificant—except to the one experiencing it.

In my own case, I had dreamed of one day becoming a scientist. It was an idealized vision going back as far as I could remember. But just as that future was about to crystallize, Vietnam intruded itself and altered those plans irrevocably. With little likelihood of a draft deferment, I decided to enlist rather than to postpone the inevitable. In the end, I was one of the fortunate ones who missed action in Vietnam . . . but it was only upon returning home that the full impact of my own dislocation began to register.

Over the next two years, I drifted amorphously with little sense of vision or purpose, in search of answers to questions yet to be formulated (a common denominator, it seems, of all forms of dislocation). Since there was an epidemic of this sort of discontent in the late 1960s, I was at least consoled in not being alone. Then, for reasons that are still somewhat vague, I made a decision to enter medicine—perhaps because, like the physician-turned-philosopher Karl Jaspers, I was "impelled by a desire for knowledge of facts and of man."[2] In any event, for the next ten years I was too occupied to concern myself with much else. All of that started to change, however, as medicine's initial luster began tarnishing, reviving once again that sense of dislocation I had experienced before. The difference was that now the desire to find answers was coupled with a better sense of the questions necessary to initiate such an inquiry—including perhaps the most pivotal one of all: that of dealing with the potential meaninglessness or (as Camus referred to it) the absurdity of human existence:

> Man stands face to face with the irrational. He feels within him the longing for happiness and reason. The absurd is born of this confrontation between the human need and the unreasonable silence of the world. . . . The irrational, the human nostalgia, and the absurd is born of their encounter—these are the three characters in the drama that must necessarily end with all the logic of which an existence is capable.[3]

In a modest way this logic has been a preoccupation ever since. Had it not been for the dislocation of that period, I might never have happened upon it. So it is, I suppose, with most adversity when amplified through time's perspective: What at first appears "like the toad, ugly and venomous," is found at last to wear "a precious jewel in his head."[4]

ONE

LETTERS FROM THE BEYOND

An odd thought strikes me: we shall receive no letters in the grave.
SAMUEL JOHNSON

IN A LIMITED sense death is a barrier to the living. To the active imagination, however, it is quite the reverse. Because of its unique ability to imagine *what is not the case*, imagination has the power to negate things. As such, it is capable of creating *nothingness* from the facts and matter of existence. And it is this concept of "nothingness"—the state most often equated with death—that creates their special kinship, and the possibility of bridging these two opposing worlds. [Perhaps Doctor Johnson was mistaken after all.]

I too have had my own secret place, a place to unleash my imagination and fantasies. This was about the time that a variety of New Age literature was beginning to appear. Some of it focused on experiences that let the right brain (intuition, creativity) outsmart the left (objective reasoning). Some of those lessons have remained with me, although they've been superseded by my reading of Arthur Koestler's *The Act of Creation*, for instance, and I had also just begun reading Heidegger.

Of course, I know underneath that these letters were a fabrication, and that I was the author, subject, and object of each, whether sent or received.

Yet I can't help wondering if there might not be something legitimate, if otherworldly, about them. Like Yeats' early poetry, the real world often seems a sad and unsatisfactory place. We are heir to this strangeness—to true otherworldliness.

November 199_
Professor Martin Heidegger
C/O University of Freiburg

Dear Professor Heidegger:

I apologize for writing at this late date. Although I've started many letters to you in the past, something always deterred me from finishing them. But this time it's different—you might even call it an anniversary of sorts.

I'm speaking, of course, about your death in 1976. (I'm embarrassed to admit it now, but when you died I was totally ignorant of the event—or that you had even existed at all!) In addition, I was finishing up my medical studies at the time and there was little time for anything else. But thanks largely to you (and a few others like you), that intellectual myopia is starting to clear—and so, this expression of belated gratitude. To be perfectly frank, I'm not at all hopeful that this letter will reach you; or if it does, that you will even be in a position to reply.

Assuming that it does, however, you are probably asking yourself: "Isn't this a little bizarre? What sane person tries to correspond with the dead?" When you've finished reading this, I hope you'll decide otherwise.

Since first taking up *Being and Time*, I've been fascinated with your ideas about *death* (and your related notions of *time* and *authenticity*). You make it plain that grasping its meaning is central to understanding the human condition. Try as I might, however, I find your concepts difficult. Part of the problem concerns the unfamiliar expressions you invented to do justice to your ideas: "Being-towards-death," thrown-ness, and readiness-to-hand, for example. In addition, my German skills are much too rudimentary for me to read your works as they were intended.

I was wondering then if it would be possible for you to write to me and briefly explain these concepts (in English rather than in German). I know it's very presumptuous of me considering that I am a complete stranger—and if you decline, I'll certainly understand. Besides my thanks, all I can offer in return is the knowledge that your help would mean a great deal to me.

Sincerely yours,
James Raymond

December 199_
James Raymond, MD
Columbia, South Carolina

Dear Doctor Raymond:

How gratifying of you to remember me after all these years. And that you actually succeeded in contacting me here is nothing short of miraculous! [I hope you won't be offended, but I took the liberty of showing your letter to several of my close friends here.]

As you can see, I am honoring your request and writing you in English rather than my native German. Frankly, I am at a loss to explain how this is possible. In life I never mastered your language, but in this new state of "Being" there is a mysterious fluidlike transformation in speech (and thought). Do not be surprised, therefore, if the style of my correspondence sounds suspiciously like your own. . . . But forgive me! We have certain rules here about disclosure, and I am coming dangerously close to testing them. So, before I get myself into trouble, let me turn to the matters you inquired about.

Death—Although I am not permitted to reveal its secrets, I can tell you this much: If asked to revise my published ideas about death (in light of my present understanding), I would alter very little. I know with certainty, for instance, that death is the only event which gives one's existence "totality." (There is nothing really surprising in this.) While alive, one's identity is never a settled matter; each moment brings with it the possibility of new choices—and thus the potential for change. Only death eliminates that freedom and permanently seals an individual's identity. This is what I mean then when I say that it imposes "totality" on an existence.

But that is only half the story. While it is easy to grasp the idea of someone else's death (I refer to this as the *third-person view*), it is quite another matter to comprehend your own (the *first-person*). When understood in this way, however, it becomes evident that death is the one experience uniquely "mine." (Other events or circumstances could have been "represented" by someone else—my job, the house I live in, etc. Even my presence at a certain place and time is not "mine" exclusively—it could have been occupied by another.) But when it comes to my own death, no one can substitute for me.

In sum, death is the only event which bestows "totality" on an identity while, at the same time, establishing the "mineness" of a life. Or, as I put it in one of my early works: "Only in dying can I to some extent say absolutely, 'I am.'"

Temporality—Let me explain my notion of the "self." Most philosophers and scientists have mistakenly centered the "self" in one's consciousness—a mind within a skull. I picture it instead as a process, an "unfolding" beginning at birth and stretching out to death. This is consistent with my view that human beings have no fixed nature, that they continually create themselves through their free choices. Yet in spite of this, human existence does exhibit certain *temporal* characteristics.

With regards to the *future*, the individual "projects" himself or herself into it with a view—consciously or not—toward his or her life's ultimate ends. He or she exists as a "Being-toward" some final goal or other. The *past*, on the other hand, involves being thrown into a particular historical and social situation in which he or she had no choice. In this respect, his

4

or her actions are never completely free. Finally, he or she is immersed in the *present* with all of its practical day-to-day concerns. But in this "everydayness," he or she is influenced by both his or her *past* (with its inherited context) and his or her *future* (with its anticipated goals).

As a result, the structure of time should not be conceived as a discrete *past, present,* and *future.* It should be seen as three dimensions occurring simultaneously. The future then is not later, nor is the past earlier than the present.

Authenticity/Inauthenticity—*Inauthenticity* results when man tries to turn away from the inevitability of his own death. To shield himself, he distorts the unity of temporality and reverts to viewing it as three separate components. As a result, existence becomes focused on the *present* while the *past* and *future* are largely forgotten. Popular culture—I refer to it in my writings as "Das Man"—is the major culprit here, with its emphasis on immediate gratification. And while this may confer some psychological security by masking the thought of death, in the end it distorts what it really means to be human.

Not so with *authenticity.* Simply stated, an authentic existence requires man to resist this distortion of time and face up to his own eventual death (I call this "Being-towards-death"). Only in this way can life's full potential be realized. How is this achieved? Usually through the unsettling experience of *dread* or *Angst:* that state of extreme anxiety which occurs unexpectedly and awakens in us a vision of our own "nothingness." When our mortality is thus confronted, we are no longer able to flee from it into the *present:* it forces us to look backward to the *past* for guiding precedents and forward into the *future* for new possibilities. Only in this way can temporality regain its sense of unity and lend a sense of coherence to an otherwise instrumental existence.

These are my ideas in a nutshell. As with most summaries, the details have been pruned considerably—I hope, however, not at the expense of the important concepts. I'll be happy to write again with additional clarifications.

Your letter, however, has raised some questions of my own. Why are you so interested in this particular subject? And how do you plan on using these ideas? I would consider it a personal favor if you would write and tell me more about this . . . and about yourself.

Most sincerely yours,
Martin Heidegger

December 199_
Professor Martin Heidegger
C/O University of Freiburg

Dear Professor Heidegger:

What a pleasant shock to find your letter waiting for me when I got home this evening! I never imagined that my correspondence would make its way to you, much less that you would actually answer it. And your summary has helped clear up much of my confusion. Please accept my sincere thanks!

You wanted to know more about my interest in the subject of death. Well . . . as I noted before, my formal education was largely "scientific." It therefore never occurred to me to think about death as anything other than a material process governed by physical laws. But when I discovered your ideas (even with my imperfect understanding of them), that attitude changed. Your view of death seemed unique to me: a key to understanding our own "Being."

Which brings me to my other reason for writing you. It is to ask your advice about an "experiment" I have in mind: one designed to test (on myself) your hypothesis that confronting death is a prerequisite to a meaningful existence. To that end, I have started to revive certain experiences from my own past; then relive them in my imagination through your perspective of "Being-towards-death." It's turning out, however, to be much more difficult than I first anticipated.

Take, for example, your idea of *Angst*. The prospect of having to wait for one of those rare episodes to precipitate an acute awareness of death would make a project like this nearly impossible. Fortunately, in researching this I came across a practical alternative: the ancient Stoics' attitude of "the constant thinking of death." To my surprise it seems to work, and I've been able to consciously simulate a modest state of "Being-towards-death" without having to depend upon *Angst* as its catalyst.

The other problem, however, is much more resistant. Thus far I have completed only one "chapter" of the project. (It concerns the deaths of several individuals who have figured prominently in my life—*third-person* experiences, as you call them.) But now I'm at an impasse and unsure of how to organize the rest of the work so that it will logically test your hypothesis.

So, I was wondering if I could impose upon you again? You've had a world of experience in organizing complex projects—your many scholarly works are perfect evidence of this. Any advice you might give me is sure to be helpful, and I would be enormously grateful for it.

Sincerely yours,
Jim Raymond

P.S.—I am enclosing a copy of what I have written thus far, so that you can see the thrust of the "experiment" for yourself.

————

January, 199_
James Raymond, MD
Columbia, South Carolina

Dear Doctor Raymond:
I read your material with care and found it provocative. (Of course, you understand that I'm biased when it comes to the subject matter.) In

any case, I encourage you to continue with your "experiment" wherever it may lead.

Before offering my suggestions—and I do have several—I feel obliged to begin with a caveat. When I wrote about death and its relationship to "Being," it was done principally as a philosophical exercise. Although I toyed with the idea of translating that theory into practice for myself, I never seemed to get around to it. (It is a personal failing which I deeply regret.) I bring this up so that you will understand why my comments must be limited to the theoretical aspects of death and existence.

With that in mind, I recommend that you follow your initial chapter with three sections, or chapters, each focusing on one of Immanuel Kant's famous metaphysical postulates (questions, really):

1) Is the soul immortal?
2) Does God exist?
3) Do humans have freedom of the will?

There are two main reasons for choosing Kant's questions as a backdrop for your project. First, because they are issues of universal concern. (Everyone thinks about them from time to time.) And second, because each question already encapsulates the notion of death within it.

Still, to be relevant to others, your project should include additional experiences of a more practical kind. As I mentioned before, however, I am not the one to counsel you regarding that. But there is someone here who is. I'm sure you will recognize her name, and her story:

Persephone was (is) the beautiful daughter of Demeter, the Greek goddess of agriculture and fertility. One day as she played with her companions in the meadows, the god of the Underworld saw her there. It was during one of his rare visits to earth and, upon beholding her, he immediately fell in love. Knowing that Demeter would never agree to such a match, however, he seized and stole her away to his dark kingdom below.

When Demeter was informed of the theft, her grief became so severe that she was unable to perform her duties. Gradually the crops wilted, livestock perished, and the oceans receded, so that at last, Zeus was forced to intervene. He pronounced his judgment: for half the year (spring, summer, and early fall) Persephone would be permitted to join her mother in the upper world; but for the other half (late fall and winter) she would return to her husband in the land of death.

To the living, of course, this story is merely an allegory.[5] But to those of us here, it is all very real. Even now Persephone is with us, and soon she will be in your world again. I mention all of this because her symbolic themes of life and death are relevant to your project.

I hope you don't mind, but I've taken the liberty of showing her our correspondence. Since my arrival here we have become great friends . . . and while I can't promise that she will respond directly, I'm confident that she will allow me to do so on her behalf. Whatever her advice may be, it's certain to be filled with insight and wisdom.

Sincerely yours,
Martin Heidegger

February, 199_
James Raymond, MD
Columbia, South Carolina

Dear Jim,

I hope you don't mind my addressing you in this familiar way. As Martin mentioned,

I do not usually respond to "outsiders" in person. After reading your correspondence, however, I've decided to make an exception. The reason is the subject matter. Death and life, as you know, are my personal themes (as they once were for Martin). The difference is that what he wrote about conceptually . . . I experienced concretely.

But let me get to the point. To complement Martin's chapters, I recommend several others dedicated to the subjects of *pain* and *suffering*. As a physician, I know you've seen your share of each. It should therefore be an easy matter to write down a few of these recollections. After that, I urge you to look inwardly at your own personal experience with them.

Why *pain* and *suffering?* Because they're the living equivalents of death and, as such, are the closest a mortal can come to experiencing it firsthand. Like death, they are beyond the body's ability to control—at times even destroying the mind's conscious contents. Thus, they symbolize powerlessness and negation. My own situation is a good example. When I was abducted, I experienced the same anguish and emptiness as someone who is tortured or terminally ill. But fortunately, *pain* and *suffering* have another side, a creative one which can carry the individual beyond them to a glimpse of . . .

Forgive me for rambling on like this. When that happens, I know it's time to close. As for my suggestions, I hope you find them of some use . . . but please don't feel any obligation about them unless you think they'll help your project.

Affectionately yours,
Persephone

March, 199_
Professor Martin Heidegger
C/O University of Freiberg

Dear Professor Heidegger and Persephone:
    For some reason your letters arrived here simultaneously. And although they're here in front of me now, I still have difficulty believing

that they're *real*. But whether they are or not (and who knows the difference, after all?), please accept my sincere thanks.

As for your suggestions, they were extremely helpful, and I have incorporated them into my plans.

On another matter, how would you feel about my using these letters as an introduction to the work? Not only do they discuss the topic of death, they also define the work's major theme: the importance of "Being-towards-death" in giving existence a sense of coherence. Of course, I realize that these are very personal, and if you object to my using them, I'll certainly honor that. Nevertheless, I think they're ideally suited for this purpose and hope you'll agree.

With sincere thanks,
Jim Raymond

March, 199_
James Raymond, MD
Columbia, South Carolina

Dear Doctor Raymond,

Although Persephone's currently preoccupied with preparations for her return to your world, she did want me to tell you that once there, she will keep a watchful eye out for you. You will not be aware of her presence, of course; nor will she interfere. (That's forbidden even of goddesses.)

But now, some unexpected news. For reasons I am not at liberty to reveal, I will be unable either to write or receive any further correspondence. And while this saddens me, I realize that it is probably also for the best. "Being-towards-death" is a highly personal matter and must be experienced in the privacy of one's consciousness. There is no place for outside analytical interference—which, of course, is my forte as a former philosopher. It is a road, in other words, for the solitary traveler.

For myself, I am grateful that we have had this brief opportunity to correspond. Whether you realize it or not, your letters have had a revivifying effect. The dead, you see, have their need for the living, just as the living have for the dead.

Our best wishes,
Martin Heidegger

PS: Neither of us has any objection to your using our correspondence.

TWO

DEATH IN THE AFTERNOON

IN *The Age of Scandal,* T.H. White describes George Selwyn, one of eighteenth century England's great letter writers and acerbic wits. To those who knew him intimately, however, Selwyn's most unique trait was his bizarre interest in death, torture, and execution. It was said that when he was not at a hanging, "his friends took care to send him a description." His interest in viewing corpses was so great (and so well-known) that Lord Holland, on his deathbed and expecting a visit from the famous necrophile, was heard to say to his servant: "The next time Mr. Selwyn calls, show him up: if I am alive, I shall be delighted to see him, and if I am dead he will be glad to see me."

Everyone to a degree (though not to Selwyn's), has a morbid interest in the death of others. Perhaps it is cathartic and cleanses us of the frightening image of our own. In any case, it is at its most cogent when that death involves someone close to us—and, in particular, when it is direct and visual. The title for this chapter is borrowed from Hemingway's story *Death in the Afternoon,* because those deaths that have affected me most have occurred mainly in the afternoon.

The Aunt

Our small town would have pleased Thornton Wilder. There were few who did not know everyone's habits and history; and with few exceptions, most people genuinely liked each other. Since it was even considered safe for children my age—I was then eight—to be on the streets alone, each afternoon when grade school ended for the day, I would walk the half-mile from the old two-story school to my grandparent's house . . . there to await my mother.

They were in their late seventies then: he was a retired "country" doctor and she a former piano teacher. Both were painfully formal which, I suppose, reflected their coming of age early in the century. Yet one could sense now and then their repressed cores of affection straining for, though not quite achieving, release.

My grandmother's oldest sister—my mother's spinster aunt—lived with them. She had been a schoolteacher and had none of their stuffiness. Of the three, I liked her best. Every day after school, she would read to me from her large collection of books which overflowed her small room into the hall and up the attic stairs. Why she never married was a mystery, and even my mother didn't seem to know when I asked her years later. Whatever the reason, it was not because she was plain: the early photographs I have seen of her show an attractive young woman with soft features and lucid eyes, outlined by thick, dark hair.

On a Friday afternoon in early spring, when there was still a hint of chill in the air, we were released an hour early from school. Instead of staying on the playground with my friends, I went directly to my grandparents' home. (I wanted to hear the ending of the story my aunt had been reading to me during the week and which she had promised to complete that day.) I entered by the side door, which opened directly into the kitchen. The old house was large and always seemed dark inside. I walked through the adjoining rooms to the parlor where my grandparents and aunt congregated in the afternoon. The heavy sliding doors leading into it were closed halfway, and I could see my aunt sitting in the large, blue-cushioned chair she usually occupied. My grandparents were standing on either side of her, partially obstructing my view.

I could tell there was something strange about the scene, which compelled me to pause at the door before entering. My grandfather looked more somber than usual, and my grandmother had a moist, glassy look in her eyes. Before I could hide my presence behind the heavy doors, she inadvertently looked in my direction and saw me there. Her audible gasp caused my grandfather to look toward me also. As he turned, I could see that he was holding a scissors and surgical tape in one hand and an unfolded towel in the other. My grandmother whispered to him and then started toward me, but he held her back. When he spoke to me, it was with uncharacteristic gentleness.

"I am afraid she is gone."

My grandmother wept quietly while he came and took my hand. "It would be nice if you said good-bye to her," he said softly as he led me into the room to see the body of the woman who was to have read to me that afternoon.

When I saw my aunt, I felt something nameless—a combination of sadness, dread, even fascination. She was crumpled up in the chair with her head bowed upon her upper chest; her entire shape seemed to conform to the chair's configuration as if she were a large, pendulous doll just tossed there. A vertical strip of white surgical tape had been placed over her right eye to close the lids, but my appearance had interrupted the positioning of the other piece. The left eye was still widely opened from the relaxing effect of death, and it seemed to be looking directly at me. Finally, my grandfather taped it shut.

Then he did something that seemed bizarre, almost comical. Producing a silver dollar from his vest pocket, he inserted it into her mouth and then pushed it far back into her throat. When he finished this pagan ritual, my grandmother handed him the Bible, which he placed under the dead woman's chin and tied in place with the towel knotted at the vertex of her scalp. She looked for all the world like an eighteenth-century painting I had seen once of a woman with a magic amulet tied under her chin to ward off the evil humors.

A month later I gathered the courage to ask my grandfather about this. He replied, "The coin was for Charon—for the safe journey of the deceased." Charon, he explained, was the boatman from Greek mythology who ferried the dead souls across the river Styx to their final place in the Underworld. By the accounts of Virgil and Aeschylus, he was a very unpleasant individual who required the payment of a fare; it was usually placed in the mouth of the dead person by loved ones for this eventuality. My grandfather said he repeated this rite whenever possible as his homage to the "mystery of death."

By the time my mother arrived an hour later, the body had been removed to the funeral home. The two women grieved and reminisced until it was time for us to leave. There was no disguising her annoyance, however, with my grandfather for permitting me to see the body. And when the time came for the viewing and the funeral, my mother was adamant about my not going because of my age and because she deplored the spectacle of the dead being "dressed up" and made up as if it were a party. "It's better to remember her as she was in life than to be haunted by that look of the undertaker's waxen art," she said. There was, of course, some truth in this. Soon, however, I did get an intimate view of that "waxen art" which my mother found so sordid.

The Asthmatic

On a summer afternoon the following year, my mother took me for a walk in a part of town that was largely unfamiliar to me. The houses there were closely packed row homes with minute front yards and little foliage. She had come to drop off some used clothing for a family our minister said was in need of help.

After we finished our errand, we started for home. We had gone only a short way when we met Mrs. L. She was about sixty, although her ivory-gray hair, sad matching eyes, and deep wrinkles made her appear at least as old as my grandmother. It was a clear, hot day, yet she was dressed in a long-sleeved black dress that seemed visibly to absorb the heat radiating from the pavement. My mother did not know her well, but she listened courteously and responded now and then as she talked.

The story of her personal tragedies was familiar to everyone in our town. Both her husband and son (and his wife) had died prematurely in separate automobile accidents. Her only living relative was a grandson whom she had raised from infancy after his parents' death. From the beginning the boy was sickly. Severe asthma caused him to spend more time out of school than in, and by the time he was sixteen, he dropped out completely. For the remaining year of his life, he spent all of his time at home in a chair or in bed while Mrs. L. cared for him. Then, three days ago, she found him dead, apparently from a severe attack. She arranged to have the viewing and funeral service in her own home, where he had been a physical (and she an emotional) invalid for all those years.

Mrs. L. was preparing for the viewing that evening, and when she suggested that we accompany her the few blocks to her home and pay our respects, it caught my mother by surprise. She stammered some transparent excuses but finally submitted while making it plain that only she would view the body. When we arrived, I was taken to the kitchen, given a glass of soda, and told to wait there quietly. They returned shortly with cheeks streaked from tears and then sat down while they continued their conversation. After a while, I asked to use the bathroom. Mrs. L. took me down the hall past the restricted room with its partially closed doors to a small bathroom. When she asked if she should wait, I told her it wasn't necessary. I closed the door, listened to her footsteps retreat, then slipped quietly out of the bathroom and down the hallway.

The room was dim, lit only by some soft lights behind the coffin. A few large ribboned baskets of flowers stood on the floor at either end of the bier. The room had a peculiar odor, probably a combination of the heat, the flowers, and the mortician's wax, that I still recall whenever I see a deathly ill child or adolescent. On reaching the coffin, I became squeamish and found myself looking away and physically covering my eyes; I gradually opened the fingers of my hands as if they were slats on a venetian blind and brought my eyes into focus on the boy's face. What I saw was neither repulsive nor frightening. Instead, it was as my mother had told me it would be: an image imitating life. Its very oddness, however, had a mesmerizing effect which seemed to hold my attention involuntarily.

The dead boy had very plain features. Perhaps in life, when the fluid movements of bone and muscle had animated him, his appearance had been more pleasing. But now those features were frozen in the awkward pose of death. The smooth plastic texture of his face, exaggerated by the dim back lighting, dramatized the impression of homeliness still more. Yet for all of this, even the undertaker's art could not mask the one thing that only life could destroy and death preserve: youth. And for as long as the minds who saw him that day in the casket existed, that image would always be one of ageless youth.

The fear of being discovered suddenly brought me back to reality from this Svengali-like trance. I slipped out and down the hall to the bathroom as silently as possible, flushed the toilet with the door open so they would hear the noise, and then walked back to the kitchen. A few minutes later my mother and I left. On the walk home, neither of us spoke, and the silence seemed to affirm my suspicion that my mother knew what I had done.

That night I did not fall asleep easily. I bundled up tightly in the center of the bed, keeping away from the edges. Even at that age I knew that fear of the dead was absurd, yet somewhere in my imagination was the bizarre fantasy that the boy had arisen from his coffin, made his way back to my house, and was now lurking in stillness under the bed, waiting only for an arm or leg of mine to break the plane of the bed so he could grab it and pull me down into his dark world below. It was near dawn when I finally fell asleep, assured by the vague intuition that the day was our world and the night his. Nevertheless, for months I stayed away from the edges of the bed until the image of his plastic face withered in my memory.

While I would experience many more deaths throughout childhood and adolescence, none of them rivaled the impact of these two images on my consciousness. It is not that the others were any less important or shocking; most of them involved people with whom I was emotionally intimate. For instance, there was a pretty blonde girl in my third-grade class for whom I felt a special affection. When she died of complications from measles, I experienced more immediate grief than with my aunt's death, yet the impact was not as profound. Perhaps her death was more of an abstraction than a concrete reality: she was at school one day and then gone the next, her passing more an absence than a happening.

The question of why those two particular deaths were so memorable remains. While there may be a perfectly good psychological explanation, there may be an even better, and more satisfying, metaphysical one. The gulf separating life and death is so wide that reason cannot peer from one side of the precipice to the other without a sensation of giddiness. It may even be that the more mature one is, the worse the vertigo becomes. Is it possible then that the very young have a clearer vision of the other side of the divide than adults because they are chronologically closer to the nothingness which precedes life?—as in William Wordsworth's "Ode: Intimations of Immortality from Recollections of Early Childhood" (Our birth is but a sleep and a forgetting, etc.).

The Corpse

By the time I got to medical school, any metaphysical considerations of death had been displaced by concrete ones. Death became for me merely a change in the body's state of entropy: from an organized array of matter requiring energy to maintain it to a disorganized dispersion of matter equilibrating with the universe. This change in attitude was largely due to my scientific education and the role models who taught me. I became, as many of the science-minded do, a functional illiterate in the humanities and its world of intelligible ideas. My professors conditioned me to be respectful only of things that could be measured or calculated and to be impatient of things that could not. One of my professors even gleefully misquoted Einstein on this subject to all his students: "A work of art or literature is for a year, maybe for a century, but an equation is for all eternity."[6] Prior to medical school, this concreteness about the workings of the world—including life and death—was mainly theoretical; there, however, it was transmuted into practice.

My initial look at death in these terms came during the first-year anatomy experience. Here a handful of students were assigned a cadaver to dissect systematically under the watchful eyes of the professor. Ours was a middle-aged man whose arms were saturated with nautical tattoos—we dubbed him "the Admiral"—and who was a derelict, from the looks of his cirrhotic liver and green liquid-filled abdomen. With the help of our instructor, my task was the dissection of the forearm and hand: to label the muscles, tendons, nerves, and blood vessels and then to point out my discoveries to my student-colleagues. Others were assigned different body parts, and by the end of the semester, our cadaver had revealed most of his anatomical secrets.

That experience had two immediate effects that, fortunately, time and reflection have muted. The first was that it caused me to view death primarily as something tangible: a corpse that could be seen, touched, smelled, weighed, and measured. Since modern science only acknowledges sensible phenomena, death is reduced to terms that accommodate the scientific model of a concrete universe.

The other effect was its direct reinforcement of modern science's central tenet: the doctrine of reductionism—the view that an accurate picture of the whole can only be obtained by breaking it down into its component parts, analyzing each down to its point of practical indivisibility, and then reaggregating the information into a scientific picture of the whole. The process of dissection in the anatomy laboratory was symbolic of this reductionist approach. Later, in courses in biochemistry, microbiology, and physiology, it was extended to the microscopic and submicroscopic realms. Nowhere during this indoctrination was the soundness of the approach challenged nor the question raised that perhaps the whole might not be a reflection of its component parts. Even during the clinical years, when we were finally exposed to living patients, the scientific approach was never viewed as anything less than the final arbiter of truth.

It was approximately ten years later when I discovered the poetry of Rainer Maria Rilke, while trying to escape the narrowness of my scientific background. One of his early poems, "Washing the Corpse," awakened in me the recollection of my own first day in the anatomy laboratory and the disguised magic in that experience:

They had, for a while, grown used to him. But after
they lit the kitchen lamp and in the dark
it began to burn, restlessly, the stranger
was altogether strange. They washed his neck,

and since they knew nothing about his life
they lied till they produced another one,
as they kept washing. One of them had to cough,
and while she coughed she left the vinegar sponge,

dripping, upon his face. The other stood
and rested for a minute. A few drops fell
from the stiff scrub-brush, as his horrible
contorted hand was trying to make the whole
room aware that he no longer thirsted.

And he did let them know. With a short cough,
as if embarrassed, they both began to work
more hurriedly now, so that across
the mute, patterned wallpaper their thick

shadows reeled and staggered as if bound
in a net; till they had finished washing him.
The night, in the uncurtained window-frame,
was pitiless. And one without a name
lay clean and naked there, and gave commands.[7]

21

By the time medical school was over, I was glutted in the scientific method and its dense mass of catalogued detail about the human body. Over the next few years of residency training, I witnessed nearly every variety of death, from the painfully slow to the mercifully quick, and the many in between. Out of self-defense, a hard psychic shell began to form—as it does with most physicians—I suppose, in order to ameliorate the impact of repeated exposure to suffering and death.

I was aware of this growing insensitivity within myself. But something else was happening as well: I felt that vague sense of dislocation returning. It was more than just discontent with my work—although that was certainly part of it. Had I then been aware of Hegel's theory of alienation, I might have fastened onto that as the cause of this vague unease. But it went even further, and as this nebulousness became symptomatic, it took on a gnawing, chronic character. As a medical scientist trained in the reductionist approach, I assumed that the problem was somewhere in my brain's chemistry—that I was probably becoming "depressed" from the stressors associated with work. A psychiatrist friend assured me that it was part of the normal "psychopathology of everyday life" which Freud had described as one of the consequences of living in the modern world. "Get away for a few days and then immerse yourself even more in your work. It will go away," he suggested.

I was now the chief medical resident, and I managed to arrange for a few days of camping in the nearby mountains. It was early spring, and the weather was almost perfect: days were bright and warm; evenings cool and starlit. After a few days I began experiencing a sense of relief; I started to think that perhaps my psychiatrist friend was correct in his Freudian interpretation.

Then one evening, sitting in front of the small campfire, watching the flames and the shadows they made in the clearing, I was overcome by the same vague unease I had experienced previously, but now its intensity seemed a thousandfold greater. At the very center of it was the distinct sensation of dread and doom: not the fear of something concrete—like a snake poised to strike—but a sudden consciousness that what I was seeing in the flames was the true face of reality. And everything I could see in it was chaotic and gruesome—much worse than any horror movie I had ever seen, and impossible to describe. I became physically ill with cold sweats and retching. When I woke up the next morning, the terror and the *Angst* were gone. Even that gnawing feeling of dislocation seemed somewhat diminished, although it was still present. In any case, I decided to cut my trip short and return to the hospital.

The Major

On the morning of my return, I came in early to review the previous night's admissions with my residents and interns. They had hospitalized only one patient, an elderly gentleman—whom they referred to as "the Major"—with leukemia and bacterial pneumonia. I decided to see him myself while they went about their other duties.

"The other doctors tell me you have a mild case of pneumonia," I said to him after introducing myself. "It should respond nicely to antibiotics and . . . I promise that we won't keep you any longer than necessary."

He was in his seventies, although he appeared anything but frail or sickly. He had a rugged build and a full head of silver-gray hair. Before coming to see him, I had looked through his record, which showed a primary diagnosis of chronic lymphocytic leukemia. But when I examined him, the only abnormality I discovered was an unsightly scar on his left thigh and some deformity below it, indicating an old femur fracture.

"A war injury?" I asked, assuming that he would have been about the right age for the Second World War. He nodded. I was curious that he had not gone to the nearby veterans' administration hospital rather than coming here. "Do you have any medical records at the veterans' hospital that we could get hold of?" I asked.

"I'm sorry . . . 'Major' may be a little misleading," he said. "It comes from a different place and time. I'm afraid our government doesn't recognize it as legitimate service."

"Where and when was that?" I asked curiously.

"Spain in the late 1930s," he answered. "I was a brigade volunteer—the International Brigades." I faintly recalled something from a distant history course about communists and fascists, the Catholic Church, Nationalists and Republicans . . . none of which I could ever keep straight.

"When I returned home, some of my friends started calling me 'Major,' and it stuck. It has been a first name to me ever since. And," he added, "my wound in that war disqualified me for service in the next."

"There must have been something almost . . . romantic about it," I said, remembering the old movie version of Hemingway's *For Whom the Bell Tolls* with Gary Cooper and Ingrid Bergman.

"I thought so too at the time—that is, until I was wounded. The sight of your own blood and torn flesh is never very romantic." He paused and smiled. "Yet, considering the current state of things . . . you're right, it was romantic." With a little encouragement he told me briefly about his Midwestern upbringing; his boredom in college and his drifting afterward; his search for a "cause" to give some meaning to his life; and his discovery of a small American contingent traveling to Paris to join the fight in Spain against fascism.

"There were about a hundred of us," he told me. "After we got to Paris in early 1937, we were trucked across the frontier. I saw a little action at Teruel, but it was the next year at the Ebro when I was shot." He rested for a moment before continuing. "I have often wondered about the man who shot me and whether he is still alive. We rarely saw our enemies, and I doubt they ever saw us. All we ever saw or heard were the small explosions of earth where the bullets kicked it up." Then he added somberly, "At least at Agincourt or Waterloo a soldier could see his adversary and feel some remorse for the killing."

"I'm curious about your injury . . . how did you get medical care for it?"

"I honestly don't remember much about it. My first distinct memory was of a dirty hospital somewhere in Madrid. A month or two later, we were back across the border, and before I knew it, I was on a freighter home." He paused again. "I suppose I should have lost my leg—or worse—but I was one of the lucky ones." He lay back. The conversation had obviously tired him.

I left so he could rest, promising to come back the next morning. That evening, after finishing my work in the hospital, I stopped by the county library and checked out some books on the Spanish Civil War, including an old copy of George Orwell's *Homage to Catalonia*, which I read late into the night. The next morning when I got to the hospital, the Major was in good spirits. I examined him briefly and could find no evidence of active pneumonia.

"At this rate, we should have you out of the hospital in a few days," I said, sitting in the chair by his bed. "What will you do when we let you go?"

"I own a little bookstore near the college. Not very profitable," he inserted, "but it's quiet and gives me time to read."

"By the way," I said eagerly, "I went to the library last night and got some books about the Spanish Civil War." I named them for him. "I stayed up half the night reading."

"You don't have much time to study things outside of medicine, do you?" he asked almost rhetorically.

"No . . . my education has been a pretty narrow one."

"Perhaps one day you will have more time," he said. "By the way, did you enjoy Orwell's book? He describes war on the front line better than anyone I've ever read."

I nodded. "Seeing so much dying must be numbing. As a physician, I even sense it myself . . . at times."

"I think," he said slowly, "that you only become hardened to it if you see it too often . . . as a passive observer. When you are a participant, you don't become callous at all." There was a pause. "It is then that you

25

begin to understand and respect death—and the whole notion of life and human freedom."

We were interrupted by the nurse who came in to give the Major some medications. When she left, he asked, "Have you read any of Camus' works?"

I shook my head.

"He once wrote that the most important philosophical question an individual confronts is whether or not to commit suicide. When you think about it—stripped of its theatrics—it makes perfectly good sense." He paused to sip from the glass of water on his nightstand.

"In my experience, most people who commit suicide are severely depressed."

"Camus did not have mental illness in mind. He was talking about rational people. Naturally it is an exaggeration, but he was referring to whether or not life has meaning and value. And if it has none, then why not suicide?"

"It sounds radical to me," I responded.

"Not really. What he is suggesting is that meaning and value can be most perfectly realized only when people face their own deaths: whether it is on the battlefield or in a lonely room contemplating suicide." He added, "For the man or woman living an ordinary life, it is nearly impossible."

"Is that what you meant when you said your war experiences made you respect death—but didn't harden you to it?"

He nodded. "When you become numbed to death, it becomes difficult to cut through the haze and see the real significance of dying . . . and living."

His comments had a disquieting resonance. I was aware of my own annealing attitude toward death. At that moment, however, something inside of me wanted to avoid the subject. "Tell me about your life after the war," I said, trying to deflect the conversation.

"I suppose I was a 'hero' of sorts on returning, but that was short-lived. By the time of the next war, those of us who had fought in

Spain were looked upon with suspicion because of our supposed socialist sympathies."

"Did you join the Communist Party?" I quickly added, "If you don't mind my asking about it."

"Not at all," he answered with a smile. "Yes, I joined before I went over to fight, as did most of my friends. I was never active though—never committed to its ideology. Yet it was one of those things that seemed 'right' at the time."

"Do you have any regrets about it?"

"No . . . although it certainly didn't make my life easier." There was a pause. "After Spain, I came back to a relatively good teaching position at the local university. Later, however, when the anti-Communist frenzy took hold, I was labeled a subversive and forced out." He sighed. "For the next few years I did menial work where I could find it. Then my father died and left me a small inheritance. With that, I got into the bookselling business."

"You aren't bitter? I think I would be!"

"It takes too much energy to be bitter—besides, it turned out to be a disguised blessing. I have had the leisure to do things I never would have done otherwise."

"What about marriage?" I asked.

"It would have been unfair to the other person. You see, I'm pretty much of a 'loner.'"

There was a knock on the door. It was a transporter to take the Major for X-rays. I promised to return later in the day, but an emergency kept me occupied. When I came back to his room early in the evening, he was sleeping, and I left without disturbing him.

When I came in the next morning, he was talking on the telephone. After seeing me, he hurried his conversation and hung up. "That was my assistant at the book store," he explained. "I asked him to bring over some books I thought you might enjoy reading—as a gift."

"That's very thoughtful . . . thank you." I glanced at his bedside chart and then listened to his chest with my stethoscope. "Everything seems fine," I said. "You're progressing nicely."

"And what about *you?*" he asked, after a short pause.

"What do you mean?"

"Something disturbed you about our conversation yesterday. Of course, that is only my intuition speaking."

There was something about the old man—a kind of congruity between the rhythm of his words and my prevailing mood—which made it very comfortable to be in his presence. He listened attentively while I told him of my vague sense of dislocation.

"What do *you* think the trouble is?" he asked when I had finished.

"I don't know . . . but there was something in your discussion of death that struck a chord somewhere."

"Your problem," he said knowingly, "is one that I am familiar with myself . . . since I have experienced some of the same feelings. When I told you yesterday that the surest way of coming to grips with your own place in the world is to face death directly, I didn't mean there weren't other ways. What you are experiencing right now is one of those other ways." He paused to let the words register. "Let me give you one example, although life and literature are full of many others. Your problem is the problem of *La Nausée.*"

"What in God's name is *that?*" I asked almost laughingly.

"Before I answer, let me ask you about something that you just brought up."

"What precisely?"

"God," he replied. "The conventional way out of your unhappiness, discontent, or whatever you choose to call it is God. Have you tried that?" he asked.

"No," I said bluntly.

"May I ask why?"

"It just never occurred to me. Besides, I don't think I believe in God."

"Are you sure it is God you don't believe in—or just religion? Don't let one poison you against the other without carefully thinking it through."

"I have thought it through . . . well . . . at least, some of it," I replied.

"But at present, you are a pagan? An unbeliever? We don't have to go into the reasons—they are not important now," he added.

"Yes, I suppose so."

"I suspected that. Since you don't have any unreasonable expectations that your situation will be solved by divine intervention, we can go on."

"You said the problem was . . ."

"*La Nausée.*" He repeated it slowly several times. "It is the title of Sartre's most famous novel, and Roquentin is its main character. He is a young historian researching the life of an obscure French diplomat. While he is trying to work, he is plagued by attacks of nausea that become more and more frequent. He eventually has to abandon his research, but he keeps a journal instead in an effort to understand what is happening to him. What he discovers is that there is no meaning or rationality to existence—and that is what brings on his attacks of nausea."

"I've heard something of this story."

"And you have lived part of it yourself . . . based on what you told me about this last year."

He was right. Some of it did feel uncomfortably familiar. "You didn't tell me how the story ended."

"You can discover it for yourself when you read it. It is one of the books I asked my assistant to bring along for you." He smiled. "Remember, I didn't promise you a solution to your problem—just an explanation."

I got up to leave. "I'm off for the weekend, and your gift should be good company. Perhaps we can talk some more about it on Monday."

He nodded, adding, "Or come in sooner if you have something on your mind you want to talk about."

Early that evening I went by his room to pick up the books. He was sleeping, and rather than disturbing him, I left a handwritten thank-you note. When I got to my apartment, it was almost eight. I hurriedly ate and then began to examine his gift.

There were a dozen books, more than half of which were expensive hardbound editions. I didn't know it at the time, but all of them had something to say about death and its relationship to life's meaning. The authors were an eclectic group of thinkers extending back as far as Plato and ending with the two—Sartre and Camus—whom the Major had mentioned during our discussions. Because of the reference he had made to Camus' statement about suicide being the "most important philosophical question," I decided to start with him. Three of his works were included: *A Happy Death, The Stranger,* and *The Myth of Sisyphus.* I took a flask of coffee and a small lamp out onto my second-floor balcony and settled in. The night was cloudless and mild, the street below quiet. By two in the morning, I had finished *A Happy Death* and then started in on *The Stranger.* As the night wore on, my absorption in what I was reading deepened, banishing any thought of sleep. It was mid-morning, the Saturday sun's yellow brightness staring into my eyes, before I finally put the second work down.

I was disturbed by the grotesquely authentic portrayal of reality in what I had read. But there was no sense of catharsis and relief in the way that Aristotle had first described it. I was left only with a heightened feeling of unease. I knew it was partly due to my own troubled nature as well as to what I had just read. The books had just thrown it into relief with their somber moods as background. I ate something and afterward slept until the middle of the afternoon. Then I started on the last work: *The Myth of Sisyphus.* Because of its complexity and essay-style, it took longer than the novels, but by late evening I had completed it. I took a short walk and then, near midnight, went out onto the balcony with the books and some notepaper to take stock of what I had read.

A Happy Death was Camus' first novel, but—for whatever

reasons—he had chosen not to publish it during his lifetime. It was of particular interest because it was the precursor of his most famous novel *(The Stranger)* and used the same protagonist: Patrice Meursault.

Meursault is a young Algerian clerk who is bored with the routine of his life. Through a lover, he meets the rich cripple Zagreus, who develops a fondness for the younger man. He tells Meursault that money is the prerequisite of happiness because only money can buy one the time necessary to achieve it. Aware that the older man had contemplated suicide because of his deformity, Meursault coldly murders Zagreus (who seems almost to welcome it) and then robs him in order to finance his own search for happiness. He travels through Europe in his quest, and when he returns to his own country, he contracts pleurisy. In a feverish state of delirium, Meursault feels curiously close to the murdered man:

> He was overcome by a violent and fraternal love for this man whom he had felt so distant, and he realized that by killing him he had consummated a union which bound them together forever. That heavy approach of tears, a mingled task of life and death, was shared by them both, he realized now. And in Zagreus' very immobility confronting death he encountered the secret image of his own life.

Through Zagreus, Meursault finally realizes that he has conquered happiness and that his death will be a happy one:

> "In a minute, in a second," he thought. The ascent stopped. And stone among the stones, he returned in the joy of his heart to the truth of the motionless worlds.

Next, *The Stranger.* In it, Meursault has "matured" from being merely bored to being indifferent to himself, to his fate, and to the world around him—all of which have a strong sense of unreality for him. The story again begins in Algiers with a note about his mother's death, which causes no ripple in his pool of indifferent emotions. At the funeral, where he is expected to show proper grief, none is displayed. The next night he goes to the cinema with a girl and afterward makes love to her. Midway through the novel, which continues to add detail to his disinterested image, he kills an Arab in self-defense and is arrested. He is so indifferent to it all, however, that he is of little help to the lawyer appointed to defend him. The prosecution takes advantage of his observed callousness toward the memory of his dead mother to show the depth of his depravity. Meursault is sentenced to decapitation in the public square. In his last hours, a priest tries to comfort him but only manages to enrage him instead (his only display of genuine emotion in the entire book):

> Then, I don't know why, but something inside me snapped. I started yelling at the top of my lungs, and I insulted him and told him not to waste his prayers on me. I grabbed him by the collar of his cassock. I was pouring out on him everything that was in my heart, cries of anger and cries of joy.

Suddenly, the prospect of death awakens him. He realizes that he is on the brink of freedom from a world that is as indifferent to him as he is to it. With that knowledge, he realizes that he is happy and probably has always been so. All he yearns for now to complete his happiness is to be less lonely at the end of his life:

> . . . for the first time, in that night alive with signs and stars, I opened myself to the gentle indifference of the world. Finding it so much like myself—so like a brother, really—I felt that I had been happy again. For everything to be consummated, for me to feel less alone, I had only to wish that there be a large crowd of spectators the day of my execution and that they greet me with cries of hate.

But it was *The Myth of Sisyphus* that was the Rosetta Stone for understanding the two Meursaults. In this long essay, Camus introduces his notion of the absurd: the uneasy relationship between an arbitrary universe on the one hand and rational man on the other. It poses the ultimate question: how to live in a world absent of meaning and order. In the first paragraph of the first chapter, he introduces the question of suicide (just as the Major had mentioned):

There is one truly serious problem, and that is suicide. Judging whether life is or is not worth living amounts to answering the fundamental problem of philosophy.

And in the next paragraph, he amplifies this:

I see many people die because they judge that life is not worth living. I see others paradoxically getting killed for ideas or illusions that give them a reason for living. . . . I therefore conclude that the meaning of life is the most urgent of questions.

Then, after defining the absurd, he outlines his main topic:

The subject of this essay is precisely this relationship between the absurd and suicide, the exact degree to which suicide is a solution to the absurd.

In a hundred pages of lyrical prose, he rejects suicide in favor of life made consequential through genuine living, thinking, and creating. This, he says, can only be accomplished by rejecting false hope (in forms mainly of God and immortality) and by substituting an ethic of *struggle, freedom,* and *passion* as a way out of despair. Camus admits that few are able to fully live life in the face of absurdity. One who did was Sisyphus, whose well-known myth is expanded by Camus in the essay's final pages.

Sisyphus, according to some, was the wisest of all mortals. To test his wife's devotion and love, he ordered her to leave his body unburied after his death. When he died and woke in Hades, he was indignant that his wife had actually followed his command. Convincing the Underworld's deity to let him return to earth to punish her, he found the earthly pleasures too sweet for him to return to the dark world below. He eluded the gods' efforts to retrieve him until inevitable death once again overtook him. But upon arrival in the Underworld, an ingenious punishment awaited him: he was condemned to rolling a heavy stone up a mountain which, upon nearly reaching the top, would tumble down again into the valley below. For all eternity Sisyphus was condemned to repeating this task. Knowing the nature of mortals, the gods reasoned that there could be no more hideous punishment than that involving futility. In the case of Sisyphus, they were mistaken.

For here is the archetypical absurd man with his hatred of death, his passion for life, his scorn of the gods, and his fate of performing a meaningless task. Camus imagines that it is during the descent into the valley when Sisyphus is fully conscious of this paradoxical joy; when he knows that his fate belongs to him alone and that no higher destiny exists for him other than the constant struggle in the face of adversity. It is here that he probably repeats to himself silently his famous sentiment of defiance: "There is no fate that cannot be surmounted by scorn." The closing paragraph reaffirms this pathway from despair to happiness in an absurd world:

> I leave Sisyphus at the foot of the mountain. One always finds one's burden again. But Sisyphus teaches the higher fidelity that negates the gods and raises rocks. He too concludes that all is well. This universe henceforth without a master seems to him neither sterile nor futile. Each atom of each stone, each mineral flake of that night-filled mountain, in itself forms a world. The struggle itself toward the heights is enough to fill a man's heart. One must imagine Sisyphus happy.

I put the books aside and looked out over the balcony into the quiet darkness of an early Sunday morning. A young couple, arm in arm, walked silently down the opposite side of the street. In another moment they were gone, leaving only the streetlights and signs as evidence of man's organized intelligence. A tepid breeze blew through the bars of the balcony, rustling the pages of one of the open books, and bringing me back to what I had read.

Miraculously, my feeling of unease had ameliorated somewhat. My thoughts seemed to be taking on some coherence, and I was anxious to discuss them with the Major. That night, sleep seemed more like a reward than an obligation.

Mid-afternoon on Sunday I awakened refreshed, with the warm sun reflecting through the window. I decided not to wait until Monday to see the Major. When I got to the hospital, I went directly to my office to check for messages. As I was about to leave to see him, one of my interns came in. He was disheveled, and his white coat was spattered with fresh blood.

"Someone told me you were here," he said. "I wanted to catch you before you got to the floor."

"Busy weekend?" I assumed that he wanted to ask some questions about a new patient.

"It was pretty quiet," he said; "that is . . . except for the Major."

"What do you mean?" I could see the concern imprinted on his face.

"We tried to call you at home a little while ago, but you must have been on your way to the hospital." He paused. "It happened about an hour ago—it must have been a heart attack or a pulmonary embolism. When the nurse went to check on him, he wasn't breathing. We tried to resuscitate him, but . . ." He was silent, then said, "I thought you would want to be informed since the Major seemed to consider you his doctor."

"Yes . . . thank you," I said distractedly. "I'm sure you did all that you could."

The intern left. I sat there alone, thinking about the Major. It was not exactly sadness for him that I felt so much, but a selfish sorrow that he would not be there to listen and talk to me again. I knew this was self-indulgent, yet I knew the Major would approve of that honest sentiment.

Then, suddenly and without knowing why, I wondered whether his death, like Meursault's, had been "a happy one" in those last moments. The only thing better I hoped for was that, like Sisyphus, he too was envied by the gods—and that they were now preparing his large stone at the foot of some timeless mountain.

THREE

EURYDICE AND ORPHEUS REVISITED

ONLY A FEW courageous individuals have ventured into the realm of the dead and returned successfully: among them, Odysseus, Orpheus, and, of course, Sisyphus. Odysseus, in his discussion with the dead Achilles, learns that existence there as one of the "flittering shadows" is a miserable fate and that it is better to be a living slave than "a king over all the perished dead!" Sisyphus, as we have seen, gleans a similar message. But it is the story of Orpheus and Eurydice that is the most moving.

It was said of Orpheus, the master musician of the lyre, that nothing could withstand the charm of his music. After the premature death of his beautiful wife, Eurydice[8], he descends into the realm of darkness to beg for her release. The Underworld's gods, moved by his music and pleadings, grant his wish on the condition that he not turn to look at her until they emerge in the world above. When they have nearly reached their goal, Orpheus glances back in a moment of forgetfulness to assure himself that Eurydice is still following; at that instant she is borne away again into the Stygian darkness.

At some point in our lives, each of us encounters our own version of a descent into the Underworld. Like all collective myths, it is implanted in our unconscious, lurking and waiting there for its chance to become personalized in the most subjective of all human experiences: the individual mythology of dreaming.

Prelude to a Dream

In many ways, my encounter with the Major and the books that he had given me were the beginning of my "real" education. It took nearly two years to finish them since they were among the most difficult I had ever come across: Plato's *Dialogues*, St. Augustine's *Confessions*, Milton's *Paradise Lost*, Descartes' *Discourse on the Method*, Hume's *An Enquiry Concerning Human Understanding*, Kant's *Critique of Pure Reason*, and assorted works by Freud, Proust, Brecht, Sartre, Kafka, Wittgenstein, and Camus. Some of these volumes were his working copies—I found marginal annotations scattered throughout. On the back leaf of one, there was even a list of books that seemed to comprise a sequential reading list—it was written in crisp blue ink and looked new compared to the textual notes which were in smudged pencil carbon. (It is tempting, though presumptuous, to think that he had devised this list as a personalized guide for me.)

As far as I could tell, the Major had been an atheist—or at least an agnostic. I was surprised, therefore, to find Augustine's *Confessions* several times in his list. It suggested, or so I supposed, that it should be restudied at intervals. The rationale became clear after reading it myself: Augustine was literature's first autobiographer and the ancestor of all authors of Bildungsroman.[9] The fact that his journey had led him to God was less important than the search itself which guided him from ignorance to self-knowledge. That he used books as his guide in this quest (in addition to God) was very telling. Nevertheless, Augustine made it clear, as did the Major in our brief discussions, that the use of books was a means and not an end—important only in its capacity to furnish the mind with the materials of understanding and to aid its thinking. But Augustine also discovered that while the rational activities of reading and study were necessary, so too were the irrational ones of emotions and feelings. For him the most painful of these urgings was his soul's scourging by the burning rods "of inexplicable fear" and "its famine of that inward food" that seemed ever elusive.

It had been two years since my encounter with the Major. My sense of dislocation had lessened somewhat over that time. Still, I could sense its presence lurking just beneath the veneer of my daily routine, like a predator waiting patiently in the tall grass of a savannah. Fortunately I had gained some insight into two of the personal elements contributing to this phenomenon: the growing dissatisfaction with my own profession and, even more crucially, the existential dread surrounding death. It was during this period that a forgotten dream reawakened, transforming itself into a personal descent into the Underworld.

The Dugout (I)

The dream appeared in its original form the summer after the death of the asthmatic boy. It stemmed from the discovery of a mysterious, deserted ballfield that my friends and I came across by accident as we rode our bicycles and explored near the edge of town. It was nestled in its own small valley off a secondary road. A camouflaged pathway sloped into its basin where, like an ancient stone amphitheater, the field lay on a steppe naturally carved into the base of a crescent hill. As we later learned, it had not been in use for nearly a decade—just after the end of World War II—because of a bizarre incident that had occurred there. My father later told me its story:

In the 1930s and 40s, before television and shopping malls, nearly every community in our area had its own amateur baseball team. Its members were young to middle-aged men from all strata of society. Our town competed regularly with neighboring communities and, for many of those seasons, managed to amass a winning record. When the war came, it brought a halt to play for the duration, but afterward the rivalries resumed.

The 1947 season began with high hopes. By late August the team was in a dead heat with its traditional rival from across the county line and one game remained to determine who the champion would be. On the day of the game, it was cloudy and rain threatened, but it seemed to hold itself back in consideration of the event's importance. When it finally got underway early in the evening, the sky had darkened considerably. After a few innings thunder was heard coming from beyond the outfield perimeter and then, as a gentle rain began to fall, flashes of lightning appeared.

By the fifth inning it was almost too dark to continue. Since the score was tied, the team captains agreed to play one final inning. With the opponents at bat, a fly ball was hit into the shallow left field; immediately the shortstop and the left fielder converged on the ball as it dropped harmlessly between them. Their momentum, however, brought them to within touching distance of each other, and as they bent in unison to retrieve the ball, a flash of blinding lightning exploded between them with Kafkaesque accuracy. The two stood motionless for a second, like stunned animals, and then fell facedown on the wet outfield grass. So quickly and senselessly had it all occurred that the remaining players were frozen in their places.

The only one who moved was the downed left-fielder, who staggered to his feet in a gesture of reflexive defiance, pitched forward again, and then was finally still. A few minutes later an elderly man sitting in the stands collapsed from the excitement and, according to the local newspaper, died later that night from an apparent heart attack. The game officially ended in a tie and was never rescheduled. It was to be the last game ever played there and, after that, the field was abandoned and left to the elements.

When we discovered it that day in early summer nearly a decade later, it was still playable in spite of the lack of maintenance for all that time. The dirt infield was tightly packed, and where it transitioned to calf-high grass in the outfield, the plain was uniformly flat. On its periphery, the faded advertisements of several local businesses could be deciphered on the wooden fences and on the flanks of the infield; the decaying wood bleachers were still visible beneath the undergrowth that had enveloped the hillside. The most arresting sight of all, however, was a solitary concrete dugout that stood on the first-base side of the infield. Its shell and roof were largely intact, and its two large doors were pulled back along its sides and frozen in place on their oxidized hinges. Inside, a wooden players' bench extended the length of the structure.

From my first sight of it, there was something about the dugout that seemed foreboding. Seeing it rising starkly from the naked ground caused an uneasiness difficult to describe: at first it was limited to direct contact with the dugout, but after a few days, the vague discomfort extended to each moment spent on the field, whether looking in its direction or not. Finally, it assumed its most disturbing dimension with the illusion that it was alive and somehow conscious of my presence and that it was beckoning me to enter.

Even at that age I knew it was a very silly phobia, but after a week I made a feeble excuse to my friends that my parents had some afternoon work for me to do. For whatever their individual reasons, a short time later the others also stopped playing there. But that did not end the matter. A peculiar dream appeared immediately after that and recurred nightly for almost a week before finally disappearing:

I was alone in the dugout at nightfall . . . presumably deserted there by my friends after having fallen asleep on the wooden bench. With only a dim, cloud-covered moon for light, I was gripped by an intensifying gloom. Suddenly the rusty hinged doors swung shut with a terrible grinding sound, and I found myself alone in a darkness. A few moments later I heard someone outside fumbling with the lock. Then the door slowly opened onto the sight of a perfectly manicured ballfield under a bright, unblemished moon. I walked cautiously from the dugout onto the infield. Nothing stirred; whoever had opened the doors was gone. Scanning the field, my eyes came to rest on several white clumps huddled together in the shallow grass on the left side of the field. As I approached, their outlines became gradually more distinct: they were the figures of the two baseball players and the old man whose bizarre deaths had occurred there years before. But now they were lying peacefully facedown next to each other. Then, with an abruptness that nearly crippled my ability to react, the unimaginable happened: slowly and mechanically each of the three arose and stood there for a moment like stone statues. Next they began walking stiffly toward me with gaping eyes and outstretched arms. The last memory of the dream was my breathless flight from these pursuers, followed by a violent awakening, coiled and tangled in my own bedsheets.

The Dugout (II)

Near the first anniversary of the Major's death, the dream mysteriously returned. The setting was the same, although time had altered both its content and its characters. This time, however, I was no longer a frightened preadolescent but my contemporary self:

Awakening alone on the dugout bench under a starless sky; the doors slamming shut; someone fumbling with the lock; and finally, the doors opening onto a well-kept, moonlit ballfield. Instead of being alone as in the earlier dream, however, standing there in front of me was my aunt as a lovely young woman—just as she had appeared in that early photograph I had once seen. She was dressed in a pearl-white robe that seemed as delicate as moth wings. Her abundant dark hair was pulled back from her forehead, and when she smiled at me, it expressed a strange amalgamation of joy and melancholy.

Taking my hand in hers, she led me silently toward the figures I knew would be lying there in the outfield. As we approached, each of the three stood up in turn. Now, however, I felt anticipation, not fear. From a distance they looked like the subjects of my childhood dream. But as we got closer, it became apparent that these were not the same three. When we were just a few steps away, I was startled by my recognition of them. Standing before me were my own personifications of death: the asthmatic boy; the tattooed cadaver; and the Major. Gradually their postures became more animated, then a sad smile appeared on each pair of lips. Without saying a word, we sat together on the outfield grass. The Major spoke first.

"Why have you come here?" he asked in a nettled yet mild tone. "We have no desire to be reminded of the people . . . or the things . . . we left behind."

The asthmatic quickly interrupted. "The Major doesn't speak for us." He looked at the tattooed cadaver, who nodded hesitantly. "He was old and ready to die. I wanted to at least live a little more . . . but my asthma wouldn't let me," he replied in a quivering voice.

I turned toward my aunt, but she had disappeared, leaving me on my own in the presence of the three shades. A brief, cynical laugh came from one of them.

"Excuses are easy," the cadaver sneered. "My life too was short. You make it sound as if we were owed something." At this, the boy looked more forlorn than before and nearly on the brink of tears. When the cadaver noticed this, his demeanor changed and he touched the boy consolingly. "I'm sorry," he said, his voice soft now. "It wasn't your fault that you died when you did. I was thinking of myself. You see, I had enough time to live; I just failed miserably at it. Somehow . . . I could never quite get started."

Something in his own words made the cadaver suddenly glow. His eyes began to shine and, as often happens in dreams, the absurd intervened. A golden trumpet appeared in his hand and he began playing, then singing, to the accompaniment of an invisible orchestra: I've flown around the world in a plane;

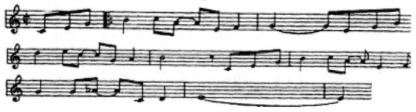

I've settled revolutions in Spain;
The North Pole I have charted,
But I can't get started with you.
'Cause you're so supreme,
Lyrics I write of you,
Scheme just for a sight of you,
Dream both day and night of you,
But what good does it do?
I've been consulted by Franklin D.,
Even Garbo has had me to tea,
But you've got me down-hearted
'Cause I can't get started with you.

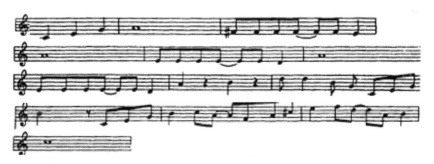

When the cadaver had finished his song, the stadium filled with the echo of applause. He bowed gracefully to the invisible audience and then turned to me.

"Why did you play that particular song?" I asked.

"Because you requested it—unconsciously, that is." He smiled, sensing my obvious discomfort.

"You mean that you can . . ."

The Major interrupted. "Look into your mind? But why should you find that strange? It was you, after all, who awakened us. By the way," he added, "my friends and I wish to dedicate that song to your . . . father."

But I already knew what his reply would be before he spoke. It had been two years since my father's death. In the last decade of his life, we had rarely communicated, and when I learned of his death, it caused little grief and no remorse. But long ago, before our relationship had deteriorated, I had felt something for him bordering on reverence. The apotheosis was short-lived, to be sure, but at the time it had seemed real enough to a ten-year old. He worked in the city then and came home only on weekends. On Friday night he usually arrived very late when everyone was already in bed. Quietly, he would ascend to my upstairs bedroom and wake me. Then, with dampened steps, we would steal to his study at the back of the house and shut ourselves in. With his record player in the center of the room and two large pillows arranged around it, we would sit there and listen to the music while he reminisced about his own childhood. The cadaver's performance startled me because the song he played was the same one that my father had used to begin and end our Friday night rituals.[10]

"That song also has special meaning for us," the asthmatic's voice cracked. "You might even say it is a theme song of sorts in our world."

"Yes," the cadaver uttered mournfully. "It is a lament for lost living, for what might have been . . ."

"Don't mind them," the Major interrupted. For some reason he seemed less bitter than his two companions. "All of us are like that to a certain extent when we first get here. It is strange, but the pleasant experiences are seldom recalled. I suppose this is a sort of purgatory where painful memories are slowly scrubbed away."

The other two stared at their feet as he spoke. Their expressions of regret were undisguised.

"If it weren't enough for us to deal with our own remorse, you mortals add to our woes," the Major declared with a hint of annoyance. "Just as we begin to slumber and forget, you reawaken us in your dreams, and then we are forced to suffer our regrets all over again until you leave us once more to ourselves."

The Sisyphus myth came immediately to mind. Instead of rolling their stones for eternity, they recycled their regrets like revolving targets in a carnival shooting gallery. "Yes . . . why can't the living leave the dead to themselves?" the cadaver whispered and shook his head sadly.

After a few moments, the Major gestured to his friends, and the three of them got up. As they stood there, they seemed to become less animated, more immobile and statuesque, just as they had been at the beginning of the dream. The Major, however, was still vivified enough to speak.

"I suppose it was no accident that you called us together in your dream. Perhaps we represent some kind of trinity for you. But there, I have said enough. It is for you to ponder . . . and decipher." He looked at his companions, who were growing ever more rigid and lifeless. "Our world is not really that terrible. Even they are becoming comfortable here," he said, pointing weakly to his friends. "None of us would ever want to return to that other world, but your visit has made them homesick. It is best that we leave."

For some inexplicable reason the image of Eurydice appeared to me. How joyful she had been to leave this somber world of the dead, and how despondent she had felt when Orpheus accidentally turned back to look at her. But these three were different: though not happy in their fate, they were at least reconciled to it and, in the case of the Major, even seemed to find some comfort in it.

"Your impression of Eurydice is distorted," he replied one last time, after again reading my thoughts. "She was not as unhappy in death as you might imagine. Your poet Rilke knew the truth."

A soft noise coming from the direction of the dugout momentarily distracted me, and when I turned back, the three of them were gone. Standing where they had been was my aunt, still youthful and dressed as before in her delicate white gown and now with a book in her hand. Motioning me to lie back and to close my eyes, she began reading to me in a soft voice. Though the words were indistinct, I recognized that she was reading from the final chapter of the story she had promised to finish on that Friday afternoon long ago. But before completing the first paragraph, I found myself asleep within my own dream.

When I awoke the next morning, the Major's comment about Eurydice was still vivid. In one of Rilke's poems,[11] I discovered what he meant when he said that he "knew the truth" about death:

But now she [Eurydice] walked beside the graceful god,
her steps constricted by the trailing graveclothes,
uncertain, gentle, and without impatience.
She was deep within herself, like a woman heavy
with child, and did not see the man [Orpheus] in front
or the path ascending steeply into life.
Deep within herself. Being dead
filled her beyond fulfillment. Like a fruit
suffused with its own mystery and sweetness,
she was filled with her vast death . . .
. . . abruptly,
the god put out his hand to stop her, saying,
with sorrow in his voice: He has turned around—,
she could not understand, and softly answered
Who?
Far away . . . [Orpheus] stood and saw
how, on the strip of road among the meadows,
with a mournful look, the god of messages
silently turned to follow the small figure
already walking back along the path,
her steps constricted by the trailing graveclothes,
uncertain, gentle, and without impatience.

FOUR

FROM ASCLEPIUS TO DOCTOR X

THE IMAGE OF the serpent has long been identified with the medical profession: the one the sign of wisdom, foresight, and prudence; the other its human personification in the physician's ideal. Two ancient emblems in particular—the Staff of Asclepius and the Caduceus of Hermes—have withstood the test of time. Though the former has come to be recognized as medicine's official symbol, the two are confused often enough to suggest that more than simple error is at work here.

Asclepius was the son of the god Apollo and the mortal Coronis. After slaying her for infidelity, Apollo rescued their unborn child and entrusted his care to the wise centaur Chiron. From him Asclepius learned the art of medicine and, in time, his fame as a healer grew. Tradition has it that he was later struck down by Zeus for disobeying him and restoring the mortal Hippolytus to life. Eventually, however, he came to be worshipped as a full-fledged god and as the "father of medicine." In art, Asclepius is usually portrayed carrying a staff with a single serpent coiled along its axis.

Unlike Asclepius, Hermes was an Olympian from birth. Although his most famous role was as the "messenger" of the gods, he was also worshipped as the deity of commerce and wealth and as a patron of merchants and thieves. Hermes, like Asclepius, carried a staff. Instead of a single serpent, however, his is entwined with two in the shape of a figure-of-eight (the *Caduceus* in Latin, symbolizing wealth and well-being). For reasons lost in antiquity, this symbol also became associated with medicine.

In light of these contrasts, it seems an enigma that Hermes' symbol should still occupy a place, along with Asclepius', in the pantheon of medicine. I like to imagine the two of them discussing this paradox in the form they would find most comfortable: the dialogue of an ancient Greek drama.

Scene One

The place: a rocky promontory on Mount Olympus; the time: the present. There is a single tree laden with low-lying fruit (center stage) with two chair-like stones beneath it. White and gray clouds shroud the sky above. The only break in their covering is a clear, sunlit area high in the sky where the distant outlines of Zeus' palace are visible (stage right).

Asclepius and Hermes, each with staff in hand, enter and sit next to one another on the flat rocks (Hermes is seated to his friend's right). Periodically they cast their glances downward where a faint undercurrent of indistinct voices originating from an earthly convention hall is heard. It is one of those large, annual medical gatherings where speakers tell about the latest advances in biomedical science, and vendors of new drugs and products hawk their wares. As gods, they can see and hear these activities perfectly, while the audience knows of their presence only through the words of the two principals and the soft background din.

Asclepius:	*(with a tone of disgust)* See how they line up at those displays like a phalanx of Persian infantry!
Hermes:	*(He nods.)* Yes! Those pharmaceutical and technology companies certainly spare no expense in attracting our physicians to their products.
Asclepius:	"Our" physicians? *(They pause and watch for a few*

moments in silence.) Well . . . I suppose it is a personal victory for you, Hermes.

Hermes: What do you mean?

Asclepius: They now worship at your temple rather than mine. The god of commerce has finally triumphed.

Hermes: Well, it was inevitable, was it not? I told you as much when we sat here four centuries ago and watched that Frenchman—what was his name?—in his study working on that thorny problem of *mind* and *body*? I told you then that the consequences would be astonishing.

Asclepius: His name was Descartes. *(Hermes nods.)* But you did not tell me how negative many of those consequences would be.

Hermes: How could I see the precise details of what was to come? Remember, not even our father Zeus has the power of foresight.

Asclepius: Still, I defy you to tell me the good that has come from it.

Hermes: Well . . . for one thing, it gave science a chance to survive and to flourish. Do not forget that in Descartes' time, the Church was all-powerful! *(Asclepius nods.)* Science was only in its infancy and might have been smothered altogether if he had not given it a basis from which to establish its own identity.

Asclepius: Go on. *(He plucks a piece of fruit dangling from the branch above and offers it to the snake coiled around his staff, but the serpent seems uninterested.)*

Hermes: By dividing everything into either body or mind, he enabled science to split off the physical realm for its own and leave the spiritual to the Church. Science had its matter with which to experiment, and the Church kept its dominion over men's souls. Everyone was happy. It was a brilliant solution!

Asclepius: I suppose, but . . .

Hermes: And consider the material progress medicine has made as a result of the science Descartes helped to create. Even you must admit that it has been remarkable.

Asclepius: *(He nods.)* But those advances . . . could they not have been accomplished without dividing the human being into two different realms of truth?

Hermes: Perhaps. *(He also reaches for the fruit dangling above and, picking two ripe pieces, offers them to his serpents, who quickly devour them.)*

Asclepius: By indoctrinating its practitioners into focusing on the body and ignoring the mind, the medical profession has become insensitive to the person-as-a-whole.

Hermes: What do you expect? Some sacred wisdom reserved for the physicians alone? You are an incurable idealist, Asclepius.

Asclepius: Nevertheless, his philosophy has helped make them callous and impersonal. *(He eyes Hermes' twin serpents for a moment.)* I cannot help blaming you a little too . . . or, at the very least, what you and your symbol represent.

Hermes: *(An amusingly pained expression suffuses Hermes' face.)* I know what is coming. After all, I have had to listen to it for countless centuries . . . though I must admit your criticism has gotten more vehement since Descartes' day.

Asclepius: You must grant that there is some truth in my charge.

Hermes: You mean, that as the god of commerce and the patron of thieves, I have somehow poisoned the souls of medicine's noble practitioners?

Asclepius: To a certain extent, yes.

Hermes: And that the symbol of my twin serpents has stamped its image onto the darker side of the profession? *(Asclepius nods.)* Let me remind you, my noble friend,

	I did not make that decision for mankind. *They* appropriated my symbol. It says more about *them* than it does about *me*.
Asclepius:	But if you had not made yourself so visible to them ...
Hermes:	Can one teach virtue, Asclepius? Even that wisest of mortals—our good friend Socrates—was skeptical about that possibility. The only answer is to select those who are virtuous in the first place to be physicians.
Asclepius:	Perhaps we could help! *(There is a hint of excitement in his voice.)*
Hermes:	In what way?
Asclepius:	We could descend to earth once again and intervene— just as we did long ago.
Hermes:	*(A look of horror distorts his face.)* Are you out of your mind? Zeus would punish us severely. Lest you forget, he forbade us long ago—since that disaster on the plains of Troy—from meddling in human affairs. *(Suddenly the heaven above is crisscrossed by flashes of lightning accompanied by the rumble of thunder.)* Now you have done it! He has heard your impiety. And remember ... he is still angry with you for disobeying him and bringing that mortal Hippolytus back to life.
Asclepius:	*(He shudders, looks toward Zeus' palace stage right, and cries out.)* Forgive me my sacrilege, mighty Zeus! It was the weakness of my mortal side that came out just then. It is under control now. *(After several moments the thunder and lightning subside and all is calm again.)*
Hermes:	*(wiping his forehead with relief)* From now on please keep your idealism to yourself.
Asclepius:	You are right, Hermes. When the affairs of gods and mortals are mixed, the results are never what either anticipates.

(Hermes nods. The two gods rise, pick up their staffs, and depart for Zeus' palace, stage right. All is now quiet except for the faint hum of human voices coming from below.)

Curtain

The Clinical Scientist

The medical school complex was situated near the summit of a long hill. From the street below, the climb appeared almost Alpine but, on that first day of school in late summer, the anticipation of the moment made it seem effortless. Instinctively I fell in step with a small group of new students who, like myself, were on their way to the school's amphitheater. After a ten-minute climb, we reached our destination.

One by one we were ushered into adjoining seats so that there were no stragglers sitting off by themselves. Soon the chairmen of the basic science departments (anatomy, biochemistry, microbiology, physiology, and pathology—the subjects that would consume the majority of our first two years of study) filed in and took their places, like privileged theatre-goers, in the first row. They were followed by the dean of the medical school and an older, distinguished-looking man in a white clinician's coat. After a brief welcome, the dean introduced the chairmen, each of whom gave us a brief synopsis of his discipline. When they had all finished, the man in the white coat approached the podium as the dean introduced him with great ceremony.

Dr. M. was the chairman emeritus of internal medicine and the most revered member of the university's medical faculty. There was something symbolic in his addressing us last, since the role model he represented—the clinical scientist—would be encountered only after we had completed the first two years of scientific indoctrination. His presence therefore gave us a tantalizing glimpse of clinical medicine while, at the same time, stressing its crucial connection with the basic sciences.

"You are a very fortunate group," he began his address to us. "You have been admitted to this medical school after a very rigorous selection process—which, I might add, has left many well-qualified individuals behind." There was a short pause. "We therefore have great expectations of each of you."

His face had a chiseled, severe expression that was softened somewhat by a crown of gray hair and a smooth, high-pitched voice. The contrast, however, did nothing to detract from the sense of both awe and intimidation we experienced at that moment.

"I need not remind you that medicine is the most honored of all professions. And while its task is a demanding one, your ultimate satisfaction will be all the greater for it. In other occupations material success is the yardstick of satisfaction; in yours, real wealth will come from knowing that you have made the human condition more endurable."

The tone of his message was well suited to the occasion, and for new, impressionable medical students, it was even inspiring. Then he abruptly shifted to the subject of medicine's evolution as a branch of knowledge.

"Our profession has evolved from one steeped in magic to one based largely on science. In between were the centuries of medicine as art— when physicians relied primarily on their experience, intuition, and personal style. Medicine still relies on these skills to a certain extent; yet it is only through science that we will attain the certainty that medicine requires." He hesitated briefly. "Do not misunderstand. I am not denigrating art, by any means. In its proper setting it is very satisfying . . . *but art without science is very dangerous as far as medicine is concerned.* And I predict that someday very soon, when the scientific model becomes as powerful in medicine as it has been in physics and chemistry, we will depend less and less on art."

The heads of the faculty in the front row nodded in unison, and since most of the students in the audience had come from a scientific background, his comments plucked a sympathetic cord there as well.

"When you finally come to the wards after your first two years," he said, "you will be thoroughly grounded in the foundations of medical science. Consider them a 'rite of passage' if you will. But *do not* treat them as a necessary evil merely to be tolerated." He paused for emphasis. "The physicians I respect the most have all been first-rate scientists."

After a few more minutes, Dr. M. concluded his address. There was a chorus of polite applause that continued as he made his way from the auditorium, followed by the dean and the other faculty. A short time later, the anatomy chairman returned to escort us to the dissection laboratory . . . and the beginning of our scientific education.

Dissipating the Darkness

The anatomy suite had the incongruous look of an abattoir hastily thrown up within the walls of a Victorian museum. Rows of metallic dissecting tables lined the center of the large room, contrasting starkly with the dark mahogany specimen cases that covered its walls. Even more striking, however, was the sight of the anatomy professor waiting there for us as we filed into the laboratory. He had a dark, Gothic look that made him seem as much at home there, among the dusty shelves and specimen bottles, as du Maurier's severe Mrs. Danvers had been among the musty corridors of Manderley. In Professor B.'s case it was more than mere allusion. He had been a fixture of the school's anatomy department for three decades—since the end of World War II when he had moved to the United States from Romania. With his thick accent and nearly perfect English syntax, he was the prototypical image of the Old World anatomist.

But it was the corpse assigned to our small group of students whose memory was the most indelible of all. As he lay there bare and gray on the cold metallic table, I found it difficult to focus on him with the detachment required of a proper scientist. The only gaze that seemed appropriate at the moment was a biographical one. The external signs were all there for knitting some strands of a narrative together, and what was missing the imagination eagerly supplied.

The corpse was probably in his early forties when death had frozen him in time. He was still very muscular and apparently on intimate terms with violence since his torso and face were crisscrossed with a series of linear scars. In addition, his upper arms were emblazoned with nautical tattoos: on the left was the figure of a bearded pirate with a cutlass in one hand and a bottle of rum in the other; on the right, an anchor with two bare-breasted mermaids perched on its concavities. Most prominent, however, was his markedly distended abdomen which, we would later learn, was the result of alcoholic cirrhosis. But striking as these features were, he had two others which stood out merely because they seemed so anomalous—these were the corpse's long, delicate fingers and his small, sensitive mouth, which seemed as if they belonged more to an artist's than to a sailor's anatomy.

"A short time ago," Professor B. said to us as we were about to begin our dissection, "these cadavers lying before you were living human beings with hopes and fears like our own. Remember this as you cut into their flesh." Then, after discussing the technical aspects of the dissection, he concluded his instructions. "You are about to uncover the secrets which the body has kept hidden from the light of day. So, let us begin to cut open your corpses and dissipate the darkness."[12]

For the remainder of the semester, the four of us assigned to the "Admiral"—the nickname we had chosen for him—labored diligently to do just that. With our dissecting knives as light-givers, we exposed his hard, fibrous liver eaten away by alcohol; his lungs blackened and cavitated from tuberculosis; and his kidneys shrunken from unknown toxins. These revelations had a price, however, and when our dissection was completed several months later, the Admiral was barely recognizable. Only his two artful tattoos remained intact. Out of some special sense of reverence, these icons were preserved by dissecting around them. It is doubtful whether the Admiral had ever received as much attention paid to him in life as we had lavished upon him in death. And in some vaguely mysterious way, I felt that this focus on him had been reciprocated.[13]

All of this seemed to demand a story—a biography—to give his presence there on our dissecting table some coherence. At least a dozen plots suggested themselves, but in the end, they all oscillated around a common set of themes: an unremarkable childhood—most likely in a small town; natural talents squandered—possibly artistic ones; ensuing disillusionment—salved by drink and drugs; escape from the world—as a sailor; and a final attempt at homecoming (or redemption)—the climax. While there was room for infinite variation in the storyline, all of them seemed to converge on a final common pathway. I imagined him arriving in the States after a long sea voyage with a spiraling illness and an overwhelming desire to see home one last time; then marshalling his remaining energy for a lonely cross-country trip; his willpower deserting him barely a hundred miles from home; and there, in a squalid hotel, writing his last note: an expression of regret about a wasted life and a request that his body be used for medical science.

Near the end of the course, I decided that someday I would try to piece together the Admiral's real history. Later, however, I came to appreciate the futility of such a search. It would be like Sartre's Roquentin in his attempt to write the history of a long-dead French diplomat.[14] Realizing that there is no "truthful" story to another's life—events merely follow one another in a series beginning at birth and ending with death—he gave it up as a hopeless task. Interpretation, not fact, is ultimately the important thing. Thus, my reconstruction of the Admiral's life was as valid as any other. Besides, his story had served me well: the names of his body parts, rather than being cold facts, had a correlative sense of history and meaning. He had helped me master anatomy.

At the conclusion of the course, a nonsectarian burial ceremony was held for the cadavers in which Professor B. gave a brief encomium. He seemed to address their spirits directly: "We stand here today in tribute to you for your contribution to our education. Although we did not know you in life, you have become real to us in death."

He concluded his dedication by reading the opening stanza of a poem by Dylan Thomas (the Welsh poet) who, like our corpse, had also died before his time. It seemed a particularly apt memorial to the Admiral:

And death shall have no dominion.
Dead men naked they shall be one
With the man in the wind and the west moon;
When their bones are picked clean and the clean bones gone,
They shall have stars at elbow and foot;
Though they go mad they shall be sane,
Though they sink through the sea they shall rise again;
Though lovers be lost love shall not;
And death shall have no dominion.[15]

The Physician Who Sleepwalked

While human anatomy was tedious, it was not the most difficult course of the basic science curriculum. That distinction was reserved for physiology. And with it came our first exposure to specialization. True to that tradition, each specialty area—cardiovascular, pulmonary, alimentary, endocrine, and reproductive—was taught by a faculty "expert." But in spite of their superior knowledge, most of them turned out to be uninspiring teachers and after the first few weeks, attendance began to wane noticeably. An enterprising student then came up with the idea of a note-taking service so those who wanted to skip class could do so. Each of us who participated contributed a nominal fee for the transcriptionist and attended at least one lecture to take backup notes in case of equipment failure.

My random assignment occurred midway through the course. It was a lecture entitled "Introduction to Membrane Transport," a topic crucial for understanding digestion and kidney function which followed it. The individual who taught that section was Dr. S., the only member of the physiology faculty with a medical degree—and a genuine knack for teaching. And since the subject matter was of interest to me because of some related research I had done as an undergraduate, I found myself willingly attending all of his lectures. Still, it came as a surprise when I scored the highest grade on Dr. S.'s portion of the midterm examination. Afterward I was asked to see him in his office.

"I was very impressed with your examination paper," he said, pointing me to a chair in his small, book-filled office. "This material is usually very difficult for medical students." He paused and smiled. "You didn't by any chance get a copy of my test beforehand, did you?"

I said no and then described the research I had done as an undergraduate. He leaned back in his chair and listened attentively. Everything about Dr. S., from his short, sinewy stature, reminiscent of an animal ready to pounce, to his cropped brown hair, raised up on his head as if charged by electricity, seemed intense and energetic.

"That fits nicely with some of the work we are doing here," he said after I had finished. "If you have a minute, I'd like to show you around."

Dr. S. had half a dozen laboratories, all equipped with the latest scientific instruments and each a flurry of activity. In one of these, I was introduced to several of his graduate students who briefly explained their projects. Although the details were beyond me, I could at least appreciate a pattern of resemblance to my own undergraduate work. When we finally returned to Dr. S.'s office, I noticed that he had spent over an hour with me.

"Let me suggest something," he said when we were again seated. "I want you to consider working in my laboratory this summer—on something, of course, related to the research you have already done."

"I . . . I don't know what to say," I replied awkwardly.

"You don't have to make a decision now," he replied. "If you are interested, write out some ideas for a project, then come back when physiology is over and we will discuss it again."

Several months later I returned with a dozen pages of notes that he helped me refine over the following weeks. Shortly after that, the first year of medical school came to a close and, a few days later, I moved into the laboratory he had set aside for my summer project.

As with most research, it turned out to be largely a series of trials and errors—especially since there was little information in the scientific literature to offer much guidance. In addition, many of these experiments were sequential in nature, often requiring my staying in the laboratory late into the evening. On one of these nights, about midway through the summer, Dr. S. appeared unexpectedly to gather some journals from his office. He had to pass my work area on his way there, and while I was finishing up my last measurement of the evening, he stopped at the doorway and stood there watching quietly.

"These hours of yours are creating quite a stir with my other students," he interrupted.

"The experiment would be ruined if I waited until morning to finish it," I replied. "They would do the same thing in my place."

"How much more do you have?" he asked.

"About ten minutes."

"I've got some paperwork to do in my office. Why don't you come by before you leave and we'll have some coffee together."

After finishing the last measurement, I hurriedly cleaned up. When I reached Dr. S.'s office, he waved me into a chair and poured some coffee for both of us.

"I've been watching your progress carefully," he said. "Judging from the preliminary data, it looks very promising. You should easily get a publication or two out of it."

"Thank you," I replied.

He sat silently for a moment, and then out of the blue he exclaimed, "Are you sure that medicine is what you really want to do with your life?"

"I . . . I think so."

"I realize it's an unfair question," he said. "After all, you still have another year of basic science before you get to the wards."

"You make it sound as if I might not like it."

"I have no right to pass judgment, of course, but I think you have the makings of a genuine scientist." He paused. "It would be a shame to waste those talents merely practicing medicine."

Dr. S. leaned back in his chair. As he did, I gazed around the office and noticed that his bookcases contained works relating only to science, none to medicine. And on one of the shelves there was an old clock prominently displayed, which had stopped sometime in the past at four o'clock.

"At one point in my own career, I was faced with choosing between medicine and research," he continued. "And watching you this last month, I can't help wondering whether you might not come to that same crossroad yourself one day."

He got up to pour some more coffee for us. For the first time, I noticed that his office had no windows looking out upon the everyday world. Suddenly, its atmosphere seemed stifling and close . . . just as I imagined a monk's cell might feel.

"Perhaps, I should try to explain," he said, sitting down again behind his desk. "When I was growing up, it was taken for granted that one day I would become a physician like my father, and his before. So in college I majored in chemistry as preparation for medical school. Those were some of the happiest days of my life. . . . And, for the first two years of basic science, I felt the same way about medical school." He paused to take a sip of his coffee. "Unfortunately, that interest began to wane as I became enmeshed in clinical medicine. What I discovered was that medical practice was based more on intuition—and mental recipes—than on genuine science. The problem with recipes, of course, is that in time they become almost automatic . . . like a reflex."

I listened attentively. Glancing again at the old clock on the bookshelf, I thought for a moment that it might have moved since looking at it last . . . as if the spring inside still had some residual tension. But I was mistaken; its hands still pointed to four o'clock.

"In any case," he continued, "after medical school I decided to become a cardiologist. Toward the end of my last year in training, I happened to be on call in the hospital one night. It had been an exceptionally busy day, and I didn't get to bed until well past midnight. Several hours later I was called to the emergency room to see a man with chest pain. I got up, admitted him, and then went to sleep again—this time without interruption. The next morning when I visited the patient on rounds, everything seemed to be in order: my handwritten history and the nursing orders I had recorded were all there." There was a long pause. "The problem was I had no memory of doing any of this! It was as if I had been sleepwalking. And yet, everything had been done perfectly . . . without my even being conscious of it."

"You didn't remember anything?" I asked incredulously.

"Not a single thing," he replied.

"And what happened to the patient?"

"He turned out to have had a mild heart attack and made an uneventful recovery. In retrospect, however, he was the most important patient I ever took care of—and also the last one. I still owe him a debt of gratitude for helping me realize what the practice of medicine had become—for me, at least."

"Your last patient?"

"Yes. That same day I went in to see my department chairman and gave him my letter of resignation. Fortunately, he was understanding, and he even helped me get a research training position at another institution."

"And you have had no regrets about your decision?"

He shook his head and looked at me as I glanced at the clock on his bookshelf. "That clock, in fact, is a reminder that I made the right choice. It was at four in the morning, you see, when I was called to see that last patient."

There seemed little more left to say. He began arranging the papers on his desk, while I took the empty coffee cups to the laboratory and washed them out. Then we left together on the elevator.

Medicine as Theatre

Our first pure draught of clinical medicine came during the physical diagnosis course at the end of the second year. After a week of preliminary classroom instruction, we were divided into fours and dispersed to hospitals around the city for the remainder of the month. My group was sent to a small private hospital in a middle-class suburb where the preceptor assigned to us (Dr. H.) had been chief-of-medicine for nearly thirty years.

Our first impression of Dr. H. was that he was too old and frail to still be practicing medicine. As with many first insights, however, it turned out to be a badly conceived one: he was elderly to be sure—in his mid-seventies—but the impression of frailty turned out to be a chimera. The longer we were with him, the more obvious it became that he used this as a guise to evoke confidence—or even sympathy—from his patients, much as an actor does with an audience. In fact, Dr. H. often used theatrical tropes in describing the doctor-patient relationship—an interaction he viewed as "theatre" in its most fundamental sense.

His own "costume" was a case in point. He always wore a dark vest with a gold watch chain dangling from one of its pockets. This prop was in constant view beneath his long, white coat, which he always wore unbuttoned. After we had been with him for a week, Dr. H. explained its significance to us.

"Time should be treated reverently," he said. "Impulsively looking at a watch anchored to one's wrist is symbolic of a world obsessed with speed . . . and it suggests to patients that your time is more valuable than theirs." He slowly removed the gold timepiece from his vest pocket, looked at it pensively, and then carefully replaced it in its marsupialized pouch. "What you saw just now was not an unconscious act. It was a ritual enacted for the benefit of the observer—and for myself. To the patient, it symbolizes the sanctity of time; to me, my conscious control of it." He smiled. "There are many little acts of theatre like that which make up the art of medicine. And when the occasion arises, I will demonstrate them."

But before showing us his repertoire, Dr. H. spent the first two weeks instructing us in the skills of history-taking, which he viewed as the primal matter of the doctor-patient relationship. In this regard, he was not very complimentary of modern medicine's scientific bias.

"The major problem with today's physicians," he began, "is that they rely too much on science and technology to do their work for them. Somehow they have been deluded into thinking that these will relieve them of their primary obligation: listening to their patients." Without warning he pointed at the student next to me. "Tell me the story of your last illness," he demanded.

"It . . . it was last winter, I believe," she replied. "There isn't much to tell except that I came down with a cold—a very ordinary one."

"Please give me the details as you remember them."

"It began with a stuffy nose, as I recall. Then, a few days later, I started to cough. Since there was some cold medicine around the house, I took it although it didn't help much." She looked at Dr. H., who nodded encouragingly. "I believe I even stayed out of school for a day or two. But after that my symptoms gradually improved, and by the end of the week, my cold was gone."

"How many of you remember reading Aristotle's *Poetics* in college?" he asked when she had finished. We looked at each other with blank expressions. "It was the first analysis of how stories—narratives—are constructed," he continued. "A good one must have a beginning, a middle, and an end. But, even more importantly, it must have a coherent plot." He looked at the student who told us her story. "Yours had the right ordering, but it was a little short on plot." He turned to the rest of us. "Your patient's diagnosis lies somewhere within that story . . . and it is your task as physicians to coax it out."

Dr. H. demonstrated this by taking us into a patient's room and eliciting a history on the spot. The patient he chose for the encounter was a middle-aged woman with a mild case of pneumonia. By letting her describe the course of her illness without interruption, however, it turned into a lengthy affair. No verbal path seemed too unimportant to Dr. H., who guided her back onto the main thoroughfare only once during the narration.

"How many principal characters were involved in this story?" he asked me after we had left the room.

"I think there were two: the patient and her illness."

"All stories," he replied, "have a minimum of three. First is the protagonist—in this case, the patient; second, the antagonist—here, the illness she is describing for us; and last, the observer—the one at whom the narration is directed: us. Never forget," he stressed, "that you are a character in your patient's story and you can therefore influence its plot."

In another history-taking session, Dr. H. demonstrated something else which he considered especially crucial: the power of fiction. We had just finished interviewing a young woman with advanced breast cancer whose immune system had been weakened by chemotherapy. Worst of all, she was in constant pain that even large doses of narcotics could not relieve. In spite of all that, she seemed optimistic and even interpreted the increasing pain as a sign that her chemotherapy was slowly eradicating the cancer.

During our first interview with the patient, she implored Dr. H. to discharge her because her condition was improving and, more importantly, because it was her "husband's wish" that she return home. Dr. H. knew that these statements were fictions: she was rapidly declining, and rather than wanting her at home, he had brought her to the hospital to die so that their two small children would not witness her death firsthand.

"A psychiatrist would no doubt attribute her comments to some kind of delusional state as a result of her disease or her medications," he said to us after the interview was over. "But to me, it is a reflection of the power of narrative . . . especially fiction."

We were interrupted by the patient's husband who had just arrived. Dr. H. walked down the corridor with him while we waited outside the patient's door. When they returned several minutes later, the husband entered his wife's room alone.

"Where was I? Ah . . . yes. Stories are a way of giving coherence to the world. That applies to both nonfiction and fiction." Dr. H. paused to be sure we were following him. "The first reflects the order of the world as we perceive it, while the other presumes that the world is not as coherent as it ought to be. This it remedies by inventing its own order." Then he added, "And if that fiction is convincing enough, it can even transform itself into reality."

We glanced at each other. Although his comments made a vague sort of sense, it was difficult to correlate them with anything concrete.

"Take the Bible, for example," he continued. "It no doubt contains some fictional stories, yet no one can deny that these have made things happen in the world. And at the other extreme, what about *Mein Kampf?* That fiction also transformed itself into reality—though a hideous one—for millions of people."

The nurse came out of the room just then with the patient's chart and walked down the hall to where we were standing. After writing a short note, he handed it back to her.

"Even in the case of our patient, her fictions have altered the world," he said with a hint of satisfaction. "In spite of his misgivings, our patient's husband has decided to take her home this afternoon. That was the subject of the conversation we were having just now. Whether her fiction played a role, I don't know for sure; the important thing is that it has come true for her."

The last two weeks of our instruction were devoted to what Dr. H. called the "neglected art of the physical examination." It was an area in which he was a master, and watching him was to glimpse a portion of medicine's true aesthetic. He began by demonstrating the discrete elements of the examination for each anatomical division of the body;

then, as a climactic, he assembled these into a choreographed whole, which he referred to as "theatre for the benefit of the patient."

"In the past, I have gotten into trouble with the powers that be at the medical school for equating this with theatre," he said, as we were about to enter a patient's room where he would demonstrate the complete examination for us. "But it *is*, nevertheless."

We followed him into the room and lined ourselves around the bed while Dr. H. took up his position on the patient's right side. The man he had chosen was a middle-aged diabetic who had been admitted earlier that day in a coma. After several hours of vigorous fluid and insulin therapy, he had awakened and was now nearly back to his normal state.

"These are the young doctors-in-training I told you about," Dr. H. said. "They are going to observe while I examine you." The patient nodded.

As we shifted closer to watch, Dr. H. moved the tray stand from the foot of the bed to the patient's lower right side. Over this he laid out a sterile green towel and placed his black valise upon it. With a subtle flourish he opened it, removed his instruments one at a time, and lined them up in sequential order (otoscope, stethoscope, percussion hammer, etc.) on the green drape as if he were a priest preparing the Communion table. Finally, he walked to the sink on the opposite side of the room, washed his hands for several minutes, and then returned to the starting position.

Then he commenced the examination. First, picking up the otoscope, he ceremoniously capped its end with a speculum and inserted it into the patient's right ear canal. He held it there a trifle longer than necessary before withdrawing it. Then he repeated the sequence on the other ear. Next, with the light from the otoscope, he examined the oral cavity, commanding the patient to "say *aahh*" several times as he pushed the tongue to the floor of the mouth with a mechanical depressor.

After returning these instruments to the towel, he then took up the stethoscope and systematically listened to the man's chest by moving the head of the instrument from one area to another. Every so often he would bring it to rest on a particular spot where he listened longer than usual, implying that his trained ear had decoded an important message from within. After mapping the chest in this fashion, he had the patient change positions several times while he repeated the sequence. When he had finally finished, it seemed that every inch of the man's chest had been explored. The patient, for his part, appeared calmer than before, as if the ritual itself had exerted some magical power of its own.

Next Dr. H. began manually palpating the patient from his head to his feet. With his hands and fingers, he systematically felt the patient's skin to detect any underlying abnormalities. His most focused effort, however, was reserved for the abdomen, where he had the patient breathe deeply as he pushed into its hollow in search of organ enlargement. He concluded his exploration with an examination of the genitalia and the rectum. Yet even this did not seem to bother the patient who by then was totally diverted by the arresting rhythm of Dr. H.'s performance.

The final act was the neurological examination. After painstakingly testing the patient's cranial nerves, his motor strength, and his sensory discrimination, Dr. H. concluded by taking up a rubber-tipped percussion hammer and tapping pivotal tendons over the elbows, knees, and ankles. Symbolic of a final catharsis, these responded with brisk jerks as if the body's negative energy were being released into the atmosphere of the sick room. After it was all over, we left and accompanied Dr. H. to his office.

"I could have gotten all the pertinent information I needed in less than five minutes," he said to us as we sat around his small conference table. "I engaged in that little act of theatre for the patient's sake."

After a short pause, someone courageously asked, "But isn't there something . . . well . . . dishonest about that?"

"I admit that there is a fine line here between art and artifice," he said, "just as there is between reality and appearance and between the mundane and the magical. And for those who are ill, the distinction becomes even more blurred—something tells me nature planned it that way."

I glanced around his office. One wall was lined with shelves filled with books. Against the opposite one was a high narrow table which looked almost like an altar. It was flanked by two busts resting on floor stands: one of Hippocrates and the other of Shakespeare. On the wall in between them was a richly framed plaque with a short verse inscribed upon it:

> Being absurd as well as beautiful,
> Magic—like art—is hoax redeemed by awe.

"The sick seem to have a special need for artifice and magic, which you, as physicians, are in the best position to supply." He sighed. "But you must decide for yourselves whether you will avail yourselves of it."

Doctor X

The end of Dr. H.'s preceptorship marked the midway point: the end of the basic science years and the beginning of the clinical ones. From thereon the focus of activity shifted from theory to practice—from the classroom to the bedside, where the measure of success (or failure) was largely subjective. And the most important of these determinants was the impression a student made on his or her resident. Pleasing this individual was paramount—even if it meant enduring abuse, one form of which was particularly common since it was considered a "rite of passage." This was the tradition of pimping: the humiliating, public grilling of a student (or resident) to test that person's medical knowledge. For the most part, it was tolerated without complaint. And with a single exception, we—or at least, I—did not view it as being either vicious or misanthropic.

I will refer to this individual merely as Doctor X to signify the puzzling, sometimes sinister, nature of any quantity labeled "X." He was a third-year obstetrics and gynecology resident who, on the surface at least, appeared normal enough. It was even rumored through the student grapevine that he was a good teacher and a likely choice to succeed the program's current chief resident. The only negative thing we had heard was that he was rigid and impersonal . . . although that was not cause for alarm since we had experienced the same traits in a few other residents. Yet nothing in these past experiences prepared us for what we were to witness in the case of Doctor X and June T.

June was one of only a handful of female students in our class. She was about fifteen years older than the rest of us and thus also senior to Doctor X. Before entering medical school, she had been a high school math teacher. It must have been a financial and personal burden because she was divorced and had the additional responsibility of providing for an eight-year-old daughter. For some inexplicable reason, Doctor X took an immediate dislike to June and hounded her relentlessly during the rotation. When it finally came to an end, the three of us assigned to him had been transformed by the experience.

"I am not here to be your friend," he exclaimed bluntly on our first day. "Whether you end up liking me or not makes absolutely no difference to me. What does matter is whether you learn something about obstetrics and gynecology. And one way or another . . . let me assure you that you will!"

The three of us listened quietly. None of our previous rotations had begun this impersonally. Still, no one was particularly alarmed.

"I have seen your transcripts," he continued. "Except for Miss T. here, who had difficulty with physiology, the rest of you have done fairly well." He paused. "But that was with textbooks and lectures; here the subjects are real people."

Doctor X went on to present the "rules-of-the-road," as he called them, in a similarly blunt fashion. We were to meet him each morning at six in the labor and delivery suite (L&D) where we would begin rounds. Then, at seven we would attend morning conference with him and after that assemble on the gynecology floor. If any patients there were scheduled for surgery, we were expected to assist. For the remainder of the day, we would accompany him to the emergency room for consultations, to L&D for deliveries, and back to the operating room for any urgent surgeries. But there was one additional rule that he saved for last in order to underscore its importance.

"We have a chain of command here that I expect you to observe without exception," he said, glowering. "The three of you are naturally at the very bottom of the pyramid . . . next come the interns, then the first-year residents, and so on. Near the top is the chief resident and, at its peak, the attending physician." He stopped and seemed to squint at each of us in turn. "You may speak to the interns and first-year residents to ask them questions. But you may *not*—I repeat, may *not*—speak to the second- and third-year residents unless they ask *you* a question first. And under no circumstance may you talk to either the chief resident or the attending physician unless I am present—and then only if one of them begins the conversation."

The hierarchy he described seemed so anachronistic that it was difficult to believe he was serious about it. Our first thought was that he was merely using it to intimidate us. But we soon learned that it was a genuine code of conduct in his department for both medical students and residents alike. Surprisingly, no one complained about it—and some, like Doctor X, even appeared to thrive in its petrified atmosphere.

In spite of the inauspicious beginning, however, by the end of the first week, we had become accustomed to Doctor X and his routine. We also discovered that our major source of learning came from seeing patients in the hospital's emergency room and then discussing our findings with him. It was during one of these early teaching sessions that his antagonism toward June first became apparent. She had just seen a young woman with vague abdominal pain, and after examining the patient, she presented her findings to Doctor X. Although her description seemed thorough, he was not satisfied.

"That was *totally* inadequate," he said after she had finished. "Worse than that, it was a waste of my time! You told me almost nothing about the patient's main problem and everything about the insignificant details of her life, which I couldn't care less about. What I want to know is the cause of her abdominal pain!"

He turned suddenly to the other two of us and began quizzing us about its potential causes. Although our answers were hesitant, they seemed to satisfy him.

"Let's try again, Miss. T. What features of this patient's pain should you have spent your time investigating?"

"Well . . . its location and . . . and its . . ."

"Help her out," he said, abruptly cutting her off and looking at the student beside me.

"Location, quality, severity, and . . . any factors that make the pain better or worse," he responded quickly.

"Did you hear that, Miss T.?" She nodded. "I want you to go to the library tonight and prepare a two-page report on abdominal pain that you will read to us in the morning. Now, let's see if you can do an adequate pelvic examination."

Accompanied by a female nurse, we entered the room. While Doctor X introduced himself and took a brief history, the patient was positioned for the examination. After he had finished, June gloved up, seated herself between the patient's exposed thighs, and began to gently insert the metal speculum. As she did, however, the patient suddenly jerked her pelvis away. When June tried a second time, the same thing happened. And on the third attempt, the patient moved her legs so violently that it caused the speculum to fall to the floor. With an impatient groan, Doctor X commanded June to move aside. He took her place on the stool and forcibly repositioned the patient's pelvis while the nurse held her knees apart. With the patient still writhing and uncooperative, he thrust the speculum into her with a single parry reminiscent of an expert fencer striking the heart of a moving opponent. After it was over and we had left, he resumed his harangue.

"I want you to add another page to the paper I assigned you—about the technique of doing a proper pelvic examination. In fact," he declared, "go to the library right now and get started on it." Just then the nurse came out of the patient's room. Doctor X stopped her. "I want you to watch this student. She is not to see any more patients unless I am present. Tell the others." The nurse nodded and glanced sympathetically at June before walking away.

The next morning June appeared in L&D with her neatly typed paper. We listened somberly as she read it aloud. After she had finished, Doctor X took it from her, folded it carefully, and placed it in his briefcase. Nothing further was said about either the incident or whether June's paper had been satisfactory. Over the next few weeks, however, his assaults became more violent, and by the midway point of the rotation, they had become unbearable for June. The other student and I tried to console her, but it was clear that some drastic action was required if she were to survive the rotation. One day she took us aside and told us of her plan.

"The only thing left for me to do is to see the department chairman. I know it's a gamble, but Doctor X is going to flunk me anyway. And this is a required rotation. It could mean having to repeat it next semester—or, worse yet, even flunking out of school altogether." She sighed. "I don't see any other way."

"Why do you think he is he treating you like this?" the other student asked angrily. "You know as much obstetrics and gynecology as we do . . . probably more."

"It's plain that he just doesn't like me," she said, shaking her head. "In fact, I don't believe he likes women in general. You've seen how rough he is with pelvic examinations . . . and how insensitive he is to women in labor." She hesitated for a moment. "I think he takes the story of Eve's curse to heart."

"Eve's curse?" I asked.

"The Genesis story: women are descended from Eve and they inherit her curse of painful childbirth." She tried to smile. "Perhaps he considers himself one of God's agents . . ."

"We would be glad to go with you to see the chairman," I offered.

"Yes . . . to back up your story."

"No, but thank you. This is something I must do on my own." There was a long pause, and June seemed on the verge of tears. "I'm sorry for that show of emotion," she whispered. "It's not so much that I care what happens to me—it's my daughter." She tried to smile. "She has been telling all her friends at school that her mommy is going to be a doctor. It would break my heart to disappoint her."

A few days later, June saw the chairman as planned. The meeting lasted for nearly an hour, and when it was over she joined us in L&D to tell us about it. He had apparently listened sympathetically while she described her experience with Doctor X. He referred to it as "very unfortunate," but stressed that it had a "purpose" even if, in this case, it had gone to unacceptable extremes. It was calculated, he said, to accustom the student to the grave responsibilities of being a physician. As far as reassigning her to another resident for the balance of the rotation (something which June had suggested as a final solution), it was too late for that with only three weeks remaining. Then, just before ending their meeting, he informed June that he felt obligated to bring this matter to Doctor X's attention. It was his duty, after all, as chairman to confront his residents with their deficiencies.

"I'm through," she exclaimed after finishing her story. "He will make my life even more miserable now!"

June was correct in her assessment of the outcome but mistaken in the means Doctor X would use to achieve it. Instead of public retribution—the torment she expected—he completely ignored her from then on as if she were a nonentity. In some respects, direct confrontation would have been more humane.

When the rotation finally came to an end, the three of us were immensely relieved. As expected, June received a failing grade and was required to repeat the clerkship several months later. This time, with a different resident, she passed. But the damage done was irreparable. Word spread along the faculty-resident grapevine that June was a problem student and a troublemaker. As a result, she had a difficult time with the remainder of her third-year rotations. It thus came as no surprise when, just before the start of our final year, June dropped out of school for good.

I saw her one more time after that. It was late in my fourth year and I had gone to eat at a small restaurant near the medical school complex. She was there with her eight-year-old daughter and invited me to join them. I tried to avoid the painful topic of her leaving school.

"Are you going to be a doctor?" her eight-year-old asked after seeing my white coat.

"I think so," I replied.

"Don't bother him with questions," she said with some obvious embarrassment.

"It's no bother . . . really." June seemed on the surface more content than when I had last seen her. "I heard that you went back to teaching. It seems to agree with you."

"Yes, I feel much better now."

"I can see that."

I looked at June carefully. In spite of her agreeable words, I thought I could detect a glint of pain in her eyes and around the angles of her mouth.

FIVE

THE SICKNESS

I AWOKE . . . AT the age of forty-five, calm and sane, and in reasonably good health except for a weakened liver and the look of borrowed flesh common to all who survive The Sickness . . .[16]

Sometimes I can't tell immediately whether I'm dreaming or awake. Then I realize it's my own heaviness which makes the world appear unreal. Once, for instance, I imagined myself as the corpse in Louis Armstrong's "Saint James Infirmary" ("so cold, so clean, so bare") and for a moment, my solidity transformed everything else around me into boneless phantoms. But those episodes are infrequent now... it takes a while, you see, for the Sickness to exorcise itself completely.

"Introduce yourselves to our newest member," Darryl commanded. The seven other people sitting around the small circle recited their first names in turn for my benefit. Then he asked, "Who wants to start?"

The Fat Lady next to me raised her hand. "I'd like to talk about . . ." she began.

"Jesus! Could you let someone else take a turn for a change?" an angry voice interrupted. "You always go first, and when you get started, no one can get a God-damned word in edgewise." The man shook his head and glared at her. "A pig at the slop bucket—that's what you remind me of."

A few of them snickered, but the Fat Lady merely glared back at them in silence. Then she slouched down defiantly, pushed back her counterfeit platinum hair, and folded her corpulent arms across her unsightly breasts.

"How does that make you feel?" the elderly moderator asked. (Darryl looked to be around seventy.)

"Like shit! How do you think?"

"Why is that? Come on . . . let's get those feelings out on the table."

The Fat Lady sulked for a moment. "He's got a lot of balls insulting me! What with his sick stories about Charlie and his friends." She turned and glowered at him. "Just thinking about you makes me want to . . . *vomit*!"

Darryl smiled, then smacked his lips loudly several times, a visible remnant of his long-ago preference for wine. (I seemed to recall that it was the tannic acid that made wine drinkers behave like persimmon eaters. Eventually it became a full-blown reflex, resurfacing even after a long abstinence when triggered by something familiar—in this case, probably the angry voices of the two antagonists.)

"How does that make *you* feel, C.B.?" he said to her nemesis. (C.B. was short for Charlie's Boy.)

"I've got a strong stomach," he smirked. "She doesn't bother me."

"You're a real asshole," she shot back. "And a stupid one at that!"

Darryl's lips were moving furiously now, like loose shutters in the wind. "*Great* exchange!" he exclaimed. "The two of you are making real progress in getting your emotions out!" He turned to me. "But now to our stories. When someone new joins the group, we go around the room and each person gives a brief biography—and then we hear yours." Darryl turned to Charlie's Boy. "You go first." The Fat Lady started to object, but Darryl cut her off. "We'll get to you soon enough."

C.B. sprawled back in his chair. Although he was in his early fifties, he looked for all-the-world as if he had been plucked from a time capsule dating back to the James Dean era. His greasy gray hair was combed into a high pompadour, and he was attired in jeans, biker's boots, and a leather jacket adorned with brass fittings and purposeless chains.

"I was about twelve when I started drinking seriously," he began. "A chip off the old block, I guess." An angry squint narrowed his eyes. "My father was a real son-of-a-bitch though—one of those nasty drunks. Whenever he got like that, he'd smack the shit out of my mother. The bastard really enjoyed that." C.B. gazed off into space. "The last time, he put her in the hospital with a broken jaw. Then he disappeared for good. Lucky for him! I was going to pour gasoline over him while he was sleeping one off, and . . ."

I looked around the room at the others, trying to imagine what their stories would be like. Then I thought of my own and what I would say in a few days when it was finally my turn. When I started paying attention again, C.B.'s narrative had forwarded to the late 1960s.

"I was living in Philadelphia then," he continued, "and the only thing I had to my name was an old Harley. Anyway, one night in a bar, I met these two guys from California. They were heading back to the coast and asked me to go along. None of us had any money, so we panhandled our way cross country." He smiled. "Sometimes the pickings were pretty slim though, and then we'd have to shake down some fag." C.B. shook his head deliberately. "Besides, it was much easier than stealing: when he drops his pants . . ."

"God, you're disgusting!" the Fat Lady blurted out. "Spare us the part about the hot spark plugs."

Darryl raised his hand. "Let's remember our rules here. Except when someone is telling their story for the first time, no one is allowed to interrupt." He motioned for C.B. to continue.

"Well, we finally made it to LA after about a month and then split up. I hustled the streets for a few weeks, but it got pretty damned boring. Then someone told me about this place out in the desert where a couple dozen people were living together on a broken-down old ranch. So I rode out there." He paused. "What a bunch of hippie weirdos! And their leader was crazier than the whole lot." C.B. leaned slowly toward me. "You've heard of Charlie Manson, haven't you?"

I nodded. *Am I dreaming again? Perhaps tomorrow I'll wake up. No! I never knew of anyone having a dream and knowing it was one at the same time.*

"They took me right in," he went on. "Charlie was real friendly and gave me flowers and a handful of peyote buttons." He grinned. "They were always chewing those damned things. I still can't believe it, but that stuff made the desert feel like it was air-conditioned."

I glanced at the faces in the circle. Although they had probably heard the story a dozen times before, everyone, including the Fat Lady, was attentive now.

"And their parties were a junkie's paradise: LSD, uppers, downers, heroin, cocaine, and God knows what else! But I was afraid of hard drugs then—still am, in fact. So I stuck to mescaline and alcohol." He glanced at me. "Trouble is, I get pretty disgusting when I'm drunk—not violent, mind you, like my old man—just disgusting. On top of that, I have these blackouts and can't remember a damned thing afterward."

"You'll have to finish up your story," Darryl said, looking at his watch.

"OK. Well, after about a week, it got pretty bad because Charlie takes me aside and says that the others are starting to complain about me. He even tells me he's worried about my health—what with my drinking and blackouts. Can you believe that shit?" He turned toward me again. "But I couldn't help myself, and a few days later they booted me out for good. I guess I shouldn't complain, though. A month after that—well, you know the rest." He paused and sighed. "Still, it's pretty depressing when a bunch of murderers think your behavior is too disgusting even for them."

Back in my locked room that night, the same nightmarish vision which had been haunting me for the past few months returned. Its Kafkaesque atmosphere was vivid enough for me to remember it in detail afterward:

As usual, I was standing at the foot of a deserted city street around dusk. The only illumination was from a series of flickering lampposts that receded into a faint blur down its long corridor. On each side were narrow row homes, all built from porous stone material and perfectly identical except for their colors. Like a kaleidoscope, these were constantly changing as a thick, multicolored liquid oozed from the pores, then flowed down the walls in coalescing ribbons. Each house was windowless; its only communication with the street being a single door around whose lower edge a razor-thin beam of light fanned out upon the sidewalk.

When it was completely dark and the streetlights were at their brightest, the occupants began to appear . . . although the doors never opened to emit them. They merely squeezed through the horizontal slits at the bottom like amoebae. Once out, however, they immediately inflated, assuming a nearly human form. But as I eventually discovered, their most unusual trait was that, when poked in just the right spot near the center of the abdomen, they suddenly deflated; then, as if by instinct, they seeped their way back under the doorsills from which they had emerged.

Soon the streetlights flickered several times. It was a signal to commence my march down the long narrow lane. As I proceeded slowly along the route, more and more of the creatures joined the procession. Yet, in spite of their swelling presence, I felt almost no pressure from their boneless bodies. Then, after what seemed like hours, I reached my destination: a large cul-de-sac ringed by brightly lit buildings. In its center stood a high dais with an ornate throne upon it.

I knew instinctively that the seat was meant for me, and I began ascending the steps with an escort of loudly dressed guards (the only ones who wore anything resembling clothes). The closer I got to the top, however, the more anxious I became. Finally, my trepidation turned to fear, and near the summit I tried to retreat, but the creatures moved in and blocked my way. It was at that moment—as they swarmed around and we began scuffling—that I discovered the site of their vulnerability. But it was purely academic, because each time I disabled one of them, another two appeared from somewhere behind me. Soon the platform was more crowded than before. At last, I submitted and walked passively to the ornate chair. As I turned to face the crowd, they applauded wildly. It was the strange sound of protoplasm striking protoplasm, and it gave the impression of a powerful, muffled wind. Only when I sat down did the commotion fade and the crowd become still.

I leaned back reflexively and placed my arms on the rests. Suddenly the extravagant veneer of the throne melted away. In its place was an ugly wooden chair. Before I could react, large leather straps snapped shut over my wrists, ankles, and chest. Then several of the guards lifted the carpet from under the chair and pulled out two large cables, which they attached to my feet. After that, four of them held me still, while a fifth approached with a bare razor, shaved my head, and placed a shiny skull cap with trailing wires on my scalp. Then the guards retreated down the stairs, leaving me there alone.

Without warning, the lights in the square flickered, then dimmed. I felt a searing pain shoot through me, followed by the tetanic contraction of my extremity muscles, which seemed to swell to the point of bursting. Without warning I began to urinate and defecate—it pooled on the seat of the chair and evaporated with a loud hiss. At the same time my nipples and penis became painfully erect; a moment later they exploded in a shower of brilliant sparks. Just when I thought the worst was over, my body fat began to sizzle, then suddenly vaporize, venting itself through the skin of my waist and neck.

As I felt myself slipping away, I looked once more into the dimness at the far end of the street where the procession had begun. I could make out a faint light which seemed to be moving slowly toward me. Unlike the immediate scene of carnage, there was something safe and serene in its glow. Before it could get any closer, however, the execution reached its climax, emptying my consciousness into a black receptacle of nothingness.

"It's the Dueler's turn today," Darryl announced the next morning. "By the way, this is also his thirtieth birthday. All together: 'Happy Birthday to you . . .'" When the song was over, there was a chorus of applause.

The Dueler nodded sheepishly. Unlike the others, there was something ingenuous and wholesome about his looks. His story, however, turned out to be even more depressing than theirs. He began with a description of his childhood and his austere family who frowned upon spirits, tobacco, even caffeine; then college where he was introduced to drugs and alcohol; next, the Air Force where his use of them increased; and finally, his brief career as an airline pilot.

"My drug was cocaine," he explained, "although I drank on top of that to avoid 'crashing'. And blackouts were my demon too," he said, looking at C.B. "To give you an idea: a few years ago I woke up in this motel room in Kansas City with a strange woman next to me. She turned out to be my *wife*! I had married her and couldn't remember anything at all about it . . . not even her name." He sighed deeply. "But my real nightmare began six months ago. I had gone home to Ohio to visit my parents, and on my second night there, two of my old high school friends talked me into going out. After some cocaine and a few drinks, everything went blank . . . until the next morning when I woke up in jail."

The Dueler's eyes moistened. The Fat Lady took some tissues from her purse and passed them to him. "Take your time," she said soothingly.

He wiped his eyes. "Although I don't remember any of it, an argument apparently started over a girl two of us had dated in high school. It's still hard to believe, but I challenged him to a duel!" He took a deep breath. "Since he was big on hunting, there were several shotguns in his truck. Our other friend thought we were kidding . . . that is, until we got to the high school football field and he saw us pacing off near the fifty-yard line." His voice quivered. "He went for the police, but by then it was too late."

"His trial is coming up in another month," Darryl explained for my benefit. "Fortunately, his lawyer convinced the court that justice would be better served if he were turned over to us for treatment first." He turned to the Dueler. "Thank you . . . I know how painful that was."

The Fat Lady took her turn next. I don't remember the details, except that she had been a nurse and a narcotic addict. After being arrested for stealing her patients' drugs, she was incarcerated briefly and then forced into treatment. The others related equally depressing stories, but after a while they all started sounding similar, and I stopped paying attention.

A few days later Darryl told his story, which many there considered the archetype of addiction horrors—not so much for the degree of the transgressions as for his persistence in degrading himself. He was also the only one there who had lived the life of a common derelict. What made this so unusual was that he was highly educated (a PhD in psychology) and totally abstinent until his late thirties. From that point on, however, things progressed rapidly: he lost his job and family and found himself homeless in the city. And although repeatedly jailed and hospitalized for drunkenness, once free he always returned to the streets and began the cycle over again.

All of this earned him a kind of privileged status among his peers. In many ways he was a modern-day Francois Villon: vagrant, thief, poet of sorts, and natural leader. True to this image, he even had his own "beggars' castle," which was constructed from an immense garbage dumpster he had pilfered and then moved to a deserted street near one of the city's wharves. There he held court for almost five years—until a particularly harsh winter set in.

According to the story, it had snowed nonstop for a week, and the drifts became so high that Darryl was literally entombed. Soon his supply of wine ran out. Then came the predictable withdrawal symptoms:

tremors, visual hallucinations, and seizures. To lessen his suffering, he reverted to an old street remedy (the ingestion of copious amounts of epsom salts) which diverts attention by creating a new illness of its own—cramps, vomiting, and diarrhea. Several days later, and near death from exposure and dehydration, he was discovered by the police. That was thirty years ago, and he never took another drink again. To reinforce his sobriety, he spent the intervening years working exclusively with those afflicted by the Sickness.

The next morning I was called upon. Since my story had little in the way of drama, I knew it would be dull in comparison. But there was no way to avoid it. Because of several "diversions," however, most of it would remain untold . . . at least in front of this group.

"It started near the end of my residency training—ten or twelve years ago," I began. "I found myself growing disillusioned with my profession." I looked around at the others. "On top of that, I began feeling that something vital was missing from my life, although I couldn't pinpoint what it was. It's hard to explain," I said apologetically, "but I guess the word 'alienation' sums it up the best."

"What kind of bullshit is that?" the Fat Lady exclaimed. There was unblemished contempt in her tone.

Darryl raised his hand. "I'm sorry," he said, looking at me. "Ordinarily we don't interrupt. Except with newcomers. I've learned over the years that they invariably rationalize when it comes to their Sickness. So we merely try to challenge that tendency whenever we see it surfacing." He motioned for me to continue.

"What I was trying to get across was that my life seemed to lack any sense of . . . cohesion."

"That's crap," C.B. interrupted. "We didn't become addicts because we're confused about living. We're like that because we didn't have any choice in the matter."

"That's because addiction is a disease," the Dueler added.

"You might be right," I replied slowly.

"Might?" the Fat Lady taunted.

"Do you doubt that it's a disease?" Darryl asked.

"I'm not sure. . . . I do know there are some who have a different view of it."

A crescendo of angry voices echoed through the small room. Darryl cut them off. "And what view do they take?"

"That addiction is more a matter of habit—or learned behavior—than a disease."

Several people started talking at once, but Darryl motioned for silence. "We'll come back to this later," he said. "For now, let's go on with your story."

I took a deep breath and started again. "For a while, chemicals seemed to give me some peace of mind, but it wasn't long before they started having the opposite effect. Soon I found myself taking more and more just to feel normal again." I glanced around at their impassive faces. "Finally, it dawned on me that I couldn't go on like that."

"You tried to commit suicide?" the Dueler asked.

"No . . ." I nearly added something about Camus' idea of suicide being the most important philosophical problem, but I caught myself in time.

"People who end up here," Darryl said, "have usually reached a pretty hopeless stage in their lives. They've lost their families and jobs, and a few, like the Dueler here, have been in trouble with the law. What about you?"

"Nothing really horrible happened to me," I replied.

The Fat Lady looked at Darryl. "Maybe he needs some . . . 'quiet time.' Isn't that what you call it? That might help him answer our questions without all the bullshit."

Darryl shook his head. "We owe him at least another session before we resort to that."

The next day I resumed my narrative with a description of my experiences as an intern and resident, including the story of the Major and the books he had given me.

"That reading kept me occupied for several years, and, like my chemicals, it made me feel better for a while. But eventually it started having the opposite effect, so that the more I read, the worse I felt." I looked at Darryl. "I'm sure it had something to do with all the conflicting ideas running through my head."

"Tell us more about that," he said with an interested tone.

"Well, one day I'd read a work by, say Augustine or Aurelius—something, in other words, that made the world appear rational and orderly. Then the next day I'd pick up a Dostoevsky or Nietzsche, and it would all disintegrate."

"He can't say a fucking thing without intellectualizing it," the Fat Lady bellowed.

Darryl smiled. "I read Dostoevsky myself once upon a time." The others frowned. Then he added, "Of course, I have no need for that anymore," which seemed to satisfy them. "I'm sorry for the interruption," he said, motioning me to go on.

"After my training was over, I decided to stay in academic medicine rather than enter private practice . . ."

There were no more interruptions, and I hurried through the rest of my narrative.

"I want to go back to something you mentioned earlier," Darryl said after I had finished. "That addiction may be more of a habit than a disease. Which do you believe?"

All eyes in the room focused on me but, for some reason I no longer felt intimidated. "Habit mostly," I replied. "Something, in other words, that we bring on ourselves."

"So we're morally weak," C.B. exclaimed. "Is that what you're telling us?"

"I wouldn't put it that way . . . exactly."

Suddenly the Fat Lady got up from her chair and pointed a frenzied finger at me. "You mean when I screwed up all my veins with heroin . . . and the only place left to inject was into my hemorrhoids (which I did gladly), that was just a bad habit?" She sat down to a short, spontaneous burst of applause.

"I didn't mean that addicts don't eventually become dependent . . ."

"But until then," Darryl said calmly, "you think it's more a matter of behavior than genetics and biology?"

I nodded. "It's easy to blame our questionable behavior on something other than ourselves. The hard part is to admit our freedom and take responsibility for it." Then I added defiantly, "No one around here seems to like the idea of personal responsibility!"

Darryl sighed. "I didn't want to do this, but you leave me no choice. We'll just have to prove to you how fragile human freedom really is . . . and we'll do it merely by *looking* at you." He glanced at the others. "What do you think, group? Some 'quiet time' for our newest member?" They all nodded. "Then, let's begin."

The room became deathly still as eight pairs of eyes locked onto me, each converging on a spot just above the root of my nose. Wherever I turned to look, they followed like a magnetic laser. I remembered playing a similar game in grade school. A friend and I had singled out a girl in our class, and by staring at her for ten minutes, we made her so uncomfortable that she nearly collapsed into tears. This present ordeal, however, promised to be a much longer one.

I glanced at my watch: nearly half an hour remaining. I tried to distract myself by looking at the wall, the floor, the fingers of my hands, even my adversaries' feet. That worked for a few minutes . . . until I again became conscious of their unbroken stares. Then I diverted myself with visual imagery: a fictional walk along the beach, the tide's waxing and waning, the seagulls diving on small fish in the surf. That worked a little longer, but when I looked up and saw their cold eyes once more, the reverie was dissolved.

The target on my forehead started to burn. Had their looks done that? Even the bones underlying the skin there ached, as if their stares were somehow capable of boring into my skull. What if the privacy of my own consciousness could offer no refuge? When the session finally ended thirty minutes later, I felt as if I had been bled by a team of sixteenth-century barber-surgeons.

The next day it began all over again, this time for a full hour. I tried another tactic: staring back. I took each person in turn and focused on that same spot just above the roof of the nose. Halfway around the room, however, I found myself becoming even more conscious of their stares. On the third day I tried a different approach. One of the keys in my pocket had a sharp point, and I pushed it slowly into my thigh. But the self-inflicted pain was neither constant nor severe enough to serve as a distraction for long. Finally I gave up. Darryl had been right. In a way they had robbed me of my freedom. I had become an object . . . a thing. Worst of all, my thoughts and my actions were no longer totally mine: they had been altered by their collective look.

"What do you bastards want?" I shouted at last. There was no response, merely immobility and silence.

The outburst, which I thought would be cathartic, actually made me feel worse. It was nothing less than public recognition of my servitude. When the session ended ten minutes later, I remained seated with my head down. A moment later I found myself alone, an insignificant point on the circumference of empty chairs. I touched the target spot on my forehead; it was tender. When I looked up, Darryl was standing in the doorway.

"After you're finished for the day, I'd like you to stop by my office . . . around seven o'clock." He turned and walked away.

"You're persistent. I'll say that much for you." Darryl motioned me into a chair opposite his own. "I'm not sure how much longer we could have gone on—it's hard work, you know."

"Would you mind telling me what you and those other sick bastards were trying to prove?" There was no effort to conceal my anger and sense of humiliation.

"I was merely demonstrating to you how tenuous human freedom really is."

"But why . . ."

"Because you gave me no choice," he snapped back. "When you said that addiction is more habit than necessity, you undermined everything we're trying to do here." Darryl leaned back and cupped his hands behind his head. "As you noted very astutely, there is little guilt if the cause of one's behavior is biological. But if it's due to bad habit, then moral weakness becomes a real possibility." He frowned. "Worst of all, they might convince themselves that they can return to their chemicals (in moderation, of course!) once their cravings are gone."

"But I still don't see . . ."

"It's simple. Most people would never get straightened out if they took that view. But if they see their addiction as a disease—like diabetes or cancer—we stand a chance with them."

"Which do *you* believe?" I asked. "I know how the others feel, but you never really said one way or the other."

"The right answer, if there is one, doesn't really matter to me any longer. But for the people it that room, it does. Their egos aren't healthy enough yet to stand the shock of taking on all that responsibility." He looked at me intently. "As for you—I still haven't made up my mind."

"So all of this was because I questioned the orthodox view of things?"

Darryl paused for a moment. "Orthodox. Exactly! You know, that reminds me of the writer you mentioned the other day: Dostoevsky. I hadn't thought about him for a long time. Believe it or not, I read every one of his novels, many years ago. Do you remember his story of the Grand Inquisitor?"

"Vaguely. *The Brothers Karamazov*, wasn't it?"

He nodded. "Although the others wouldn't approve, it's one of my favorites." Darryl opened the top drawer of his desk and removed a copy of the forbidden book. "It begins with Christ's return to earth at the time of the Spanish Inquisition. The Grand Inquisitor finds out about it and has him seized. That same evening he visits him in prison and explains why he can't allow him to resume his ministry." He began reading:

What message did you preach in Palestine? That all men must strive for more abundant life, that they should not be content to be mere men. You raised the standard of conduct. Then you left us to build a Church on your precepts. What you didn't seem to realize is that all men are not moral geniuses. It is not the Church's business to save only those few who are strong-willed enough to save themselves. We are concerned about raising the general standard of the race, and we can't do this by telling every man that he had better be his own Church—as you did. You raised the standard too high, and we have had to haul it down again. We, the elect, are unhappy—because we know just how terribly difficult it is to "achieve salvation." But we have always kept this secret from the people—who are not much better than dogs and cats, after all. Now you come back, proposing to give the show away! Do you suppose I can allow that? I am afraid I shall have to have you quietly done away with and it is entirely your own fault. Prophets are all very well when they are dead, but while they are alive there is nothing for it but to burn or crucify them.[17]

"I suppose that over the years I have become a Grand Inquisitor of sorts," he said, returning the book to the drawer. "Like him, I've tried to protect my flock from the unorthodox—for their own sake, of course." He sighed. "In any case, I want to thank you for reminding me of my own burden." He arose and reached out his hand. "I think it would be a good idea if we had a few more of these sessions. Who knows? You may even become one of the 'faithful' yourself."

"Yes, I'd like that," I replied.

The next morning the fast of silence was officially broken. I was not called upon since the others had accumulated a backlog of issues over the three days of my ordeal. For some reason, their monologues sounded even more masochistic and self-derogatory than before. I asked Darryl about it when we met later that evening.

"Why do they seem to enjoy degrading themselves so much?"

"Because it gets to the heart of the matter," he replied. "Reliving those past horrors is the best deterrent there is to repeating them." He leaned back. "It's also a social phenomenon. You've probably noticed our little hierarchy here . . . where the worst offenders are accorded the greatest respect?"

I nodded.

"But getting that personal garbage out in the open is only the first step. Their egos still need to be deflated. Only after that is done can we start to rebuild them."

"How do you do that—deflate their egos, I mean?"

"It's simple. You 'infantize' them—make them dependent upon you, as if they were small children."

"That doesn't sound so simple to me."

"It's not nearly as difficult as you might imagine. You begin by destroying all of their statements about themselves. You've already seen it at work here . . . on yourself." Darryl leaned back. "Have you ever heard the term 'discourse of power'?"[18]

"I'm not sure . . . I don't think so."

"It refers to the fact that every group in society evolves a unique language (or discourse) which it uses to its own advantage. To become a member of that group, a person has to first go through special training to become fluent in it." He pointed to a medical dictionary lying on the desk. "Your own profession is a perfect example. It confers power because only another physician can understand it fully."

"And what language do you use here?" I asked.

"Ours is a hybrid of sorts. We borrow terms from psychiatry, psychology, sociology . . . even religion." He leaned forward. "Do you remember when the Fat Lady accused you of intellectualizing?" I nodded. "You probably didn't realize it then, but when that accusation was made, you were already doomed. That's because each time you counter it with a logical argument, the argument itself becomes subject to the charge." Darryl smiled. "So you see, in the end there's no place to run for cover."

"It sounds more like a parlor game than an attempt to help someone."

"Perhaps . . . but with addicts the results are more important than the means." Darryl looked at his watch. "We'll have to end a little early tonight, and I want to ask a favor of you. Tomorrow I want you to tell the group something shocking about yourself."

"But . . . why?"

"Because it might help break the ice and get them off your back."

"What if I don't have anything to tell?"

"Then invent something that *might* have been."

"You mean *lie?*"

"I don't consider a little creative rearranging of the facts to be lying. It's storytelling—and besides, there's some truth in every story."

Darryl got up from behind his desk and walked me to the door. As he opened it, I turned and stood there for a moment.

"Why are you telling me all of this? Aren't you giving away secrets?"

He smiled. "Even a Grand Inquisitor has to rest from his duties now and then."

The next morning the Fat Lady asked to go first. She was visibly agitated by a dream from the previous night—one of those familiar relapse visions that every addict experiences early in recovery.

"I was back in my apartment," she began, "with two of my old friends. One of them had enough heroin to keep us for a month. The only problem was that we were locked in—from the outside—and no one had any syringes." She took a deep breath. "It was like dying of thirst in the desert with a water hole in sight and not being able to get to it."

"What do you think your dream is trying to tell you?" Darryl asked.

"That I'm getting ready to use again?"

He shook his head. "I believe it's telling you that even if your drugs were available, something inside you would still say no."

"Especially since there's another way of giving yourself heroin," I interrupted. It was my first unsolicited comment since the ordeal of silence, and everyone glared at me.

"What do you know about it?" the Fat Lady blurted out.

"Let him talk," Darryl said, turning to me.

"It's the old pin and dropper method . . ."

"How the fuck do you get *that* into a vein?" C.B. exclaimed.

"You don't put it *into* a vein," I replied condescendingly. "You squeeze up some flesh on your thigh, then take a pin and stab it. After that, you put the dropper *over* the hole and let it in slowly under a little pressure." I looked around at each of them. "Besides, it's safer than mainlining."

"Safer?" C.B. repeated.

"It's easier to give yourself a test dose that way—and you might even avoid a 'loaded' one." There were blank looks all around the circle. "Heroin that's been poisoned," I added.

"Why would anybody do that?" the Dueler asked.

"It's the easiest way to get rid of a junkie who's become a real pain in the ass. The supplier just mixes a little strychnine in with the heroin. After all, they look exactly alike." Everyone sat up attentively. "I only saw it once—and it worked so fast that the poor bastard didn't have enough time to pull the needle out of his arm. The moment the stuff was in, his jaw clamped shut and he slumped over." I leaned back. "The needle was still dangling from his arm—like a ripe pear—when the police found him."[19]

Everyone was perfectly still. When I looked at Darryl, I could see that he was concealing an impatient smile.

"Another performance like that and they'll soon accept you as one of their own," he said to me that evening. "I won't ask, of course, whether it was true or not."

"Still, I feel a little guilty."

"There's no need to," he replied. "Your obligation right now is to yourself. You must do whatever it takes to get through this—even if that means bending the truth at times. And since you're going to be here for another month, let's try to make the most out of it by continuing these evening sessions."

I agreed, and for the rest of my time there we met every evening in his small office. There was no agenda and no topic was considered off-limits or too trivial to discuss. But it wasn't until the end of my last week there that the subject of death finally came up.

"It seems to me," Darryl said, "that many of the important events in your life have been associated with the idea of death." He leaned toward me. "And whether you realize it or not, even your presence here is connected with that theme—in this case, your own death."

"What do you mean?"

"Well, the Sickness makes you realize how powerless you really are. And isn't that the epitome of death? It's the one event no human being has any control over—unless, of course, you chose suicide." He looked at me intently. "And when that realization becomes intense enough, it can have a transforming effect."

"Have you ever had that kind of experience?" I asked.

He nodded. "It was during that snowstorm thirty years ago. That was the one time in my life I was truly convinced I was going to die. You know, it's funny how time loses all sense of motion when you sense that death is near. It slows to a snail's pace . . ." I glanced at Darryl's face; for a moment it appeared almost youthful. "Then, as I was slipping into unconsciousness, I had this eerie feeling that something—or someone—was present. I managed to prop myself up and saw this strange light approaching from somewhere near my feet." He leaned back in his chair. "There was something so completely serene about it that I knew everything would be fine from then on. The next thing I remember was waking up in a hospital bed."

I'm not sure why I hadn't thought of it before, but suddenly the image of that recurrent nightmare flashed in front of me. Like Darryl's vision, it too had culminated in the approach of a mysterious, comforting light.

"You look preoccupied," he said.

"There's something I haven't mentioned before . . . and it may be important." I described the dream for him, and afterward Darryl sat silently for a time.

"Perhaps," he said at last, "you were on the verge of an experience like mine. But for some reason your dream wasn't a strong enough stimulus to push you over the threshold." Then with a pitch of excitement, he said, "I want you to think about something for me tonight. And since you'll be leaving this place in a few days, I'll need your answer *tomorrow*."

"What is it?" I asked.

"In all those experiences of death you told me about, you always played the role of a passive observer. *Except* for your nightmare—and that one time in the mountains when you had an encounter with *Angst*." Darryl leaned toward me. "I want you to try and remember another one you might have forgotten: one where the ordeal of death is again your own." He sat back once more. "It might provide a link to your recent dream—and be the additional catalyst you need."

"But don't you think I would have remembered something like that?"

"I don't know . . . maybe it's weighted down under years of other memories. Just promise me you'll try."

"I will."

That night I stayed awake struggling to dislodge that fragment of memory. As invariably happens, however, the harder I tried, the more unyielding my efforts became. Finally around dawn I gave up. Just as I was dozing off, a dog began to bark in the distance and, in a miraculous surge, the images appeared in rapid succession. After that I slept soundly for several hours. When I walked into Darryl's office that evening, he was brimming with anticipation.

"Well, what did you discover?" he asked.

"I'm not sure it's what you asked for, but under the circumstances, it's the best I could do." I described how the dog's barking had set off a chain of associations.

"Go on."

"Which, in turn, reminded me of its setting: a camp on the outskirts of the valley where I grew up. When I was a boy, my parents sent me there for two or three summers. It's amazing," I exclaimed, "how a memory can lie buried for all that time and then resurface so clearly—as if it happened only yesterday."

Darryl nodded.

"But the thing I remember most about it were the Saturday night campfires . . . and the stories the counselors told us as we huddled together in the dark. One counselor, in particular, stands out in my mind. He was part Indian and, on top of that, his ancestors—the Leni Lenape—had been the original inhabitants of the area." I paused for a moment to catch my breath.

"Unlike the others, his stories always sounded real. One that I recall, in particular, was about a small valley hidden somewhere within the borders of camp. The legend went that the Sun God had created it by uprooting a sacred tree that grew there—a gigantic oak joining heaven and earth to the Underworld. There was also a large cave there which had been formed from the tree's central root. And this tunnel led directly into the lower world where the spirits of the dead resided."

I stopped for a moment while Darryl got up to pour us each some coffee. "That story sounds vaguely familiar," he said as he sat down again. "But I didn't mean to interrupt you—go on."

"Because of its sacred nature, the valley was used by the tribe in their initiation rites. When an Indian boy turned twelve, for example, the elders would take him into the valley and leave him there alone for three or four days." I took a sip of coffee. "He never told us exactly what happened to the boys, except that they were expected to enter the cave and confront the spirits of the dead."

There was a pause. "How much of his story do you believe?" he finally asked.

"I'm not sure, but he swore the valley was a real place. He even told us that he had been there several times himself." I paused for a moment. "I know it's not exactly what you had asked for."

He shook his head. "As a matter of fact, I think it's perfect! It may turn out to be just the catalyst you need." He tipped forward in his chair. "Now that you've reawakened all of this, don't you have an obligation to search out the reality behind it?"

"You mean, look for it myself? But, I'm not sure how . . . or when I'd find the time."

Darryl smiled omnisciently. "I think you will, however. And when you do, be sure to record your experiences in a journal. You can never tell . . . it might come in handy someday."

"I'll certainly think about it."

"You know, I really envy you," he said with a sigh. "The chance of finding something like that doesn't come around very often—especially since the world frowns upon hidden places." Darryl stood up. "You'll let me know about your progress, won't you? And promise that you'll keep the other things you learned here in mind."

"I will . . . and thank you. I mean that sincerely." Then we said goodbye for the last time.

SIX

THE SEPULCHER OF GOD

WHEN FRIEDRICH NIETZSCHE announced the "death of God" over a century ago, he considered it the most significant event in the long expanse of human history. With brilliant irony, Nietzsche decided upon a madman to herald his unbelievable truth:

> Have you not heard of that madman who lit a lantern in the bright morning hours, ran to the market place, and cried incessantly, "I seek God! I seek God!" As many of those who do not believe in God were standing around just then, he provoked much laughter. Why, did he get lost? said one. Did he lose his way like a child? said another. . . . The madman jumped into their midst and pierced them with his glances.
> "Whither is God?" he cried. "I shall tell you. *We have killed him*—you and I. All of us are his murderers. But how have we done this? How were we able to drink up the sea? Who gave us the sponge to wipe away the entire horizon. . . . Must not lanterns be lit in the morning? Do we not hear anything yet of the noise of the gravediggers who are burying God? Do we not smell anything yet of God's decomposition. . . . God is dead. God remains dead. And we have killed him. How shall we, the murderers of all murderers, comfort ourselves? . . . Who will wipe this blood off us?[20]

For Nietzsche this was a liberating event. But for many of us today, it evokes an inescapable sense of nostalgia for that which has been ir-retrievably lost.

Trinity

The main characters in my dugout dream were a "kind of trinity"—one whose meaning was left for me to decipher. On the surface, at least, the three of them appeared to symbolize youth, maturity, and old age (or past, present, and future). But further down, beneath the superficial ap-pearances, was another level in which were embedded the transmitted metaphors of my own inherited religious tradition: in particular, the image of the Holy Trinity. It was only natural, then, that it would even-tually lead me to an examination of my own religious beliefs which, like the object of investigation, disclosed a triad of its own—although, in this case, a developmental one: beginning from a stage of uncriti-cal acceptance (ingenuousness), through one of doubt (skepticism), to variable insight.[21]

Ingenuousness

My earliest memory of formal religion is of a large gathering of small children on a long-ago Sunday morning near Christmastime in the basement of our Lutheran church while, somewhere in its corpus above us, the adults worshiped free from our distractions. Its surrealistic imag-es are still distinct: a large room full of low tables, each with a miniature tree covered in ornaments resembling birds; a throng of noisy children, myself included, sitting around them; smiling matrons sipping coffee and distributing a small picture of the Bethlehem manger scene and a quartered orange to each of us; the juice trickling from our mouths onto the pictures of the Christ child; and finally the matrons attempt-ing to wipe the glutinous surfaces of the pictures clean but ruining them instead.

Wallace Stevens, born before the turn of the century in the next valley over from our own, wrote a poem in 1923 of the same name.[22]

Whenever I hear it now, it evokes the special contentment of that early imagery while foreshadowing the more somber realities to come.

Complacencies of the peignoir, and late
Coffee and oranges in a sunny chair,
And the green freedom of a cockatoo
Upon a rug mingle to dissipate
The holy hush of ancient sacrifice.
She dreams a little, and she feels the dark
Encroachment of that old catastrophe,
As a calm darkens among water-lights.
The pungent oranges and bright, green wings
Seem things in some procession of the dead,
Winding across wide water, without sound.
The day is like wide water, without sound,
Stilled for the passing of her dreaming feet
Over the seas, to silent Palestine,
Dominion of the blood and sepulchre.

Conventional Lutheranism was only one hemisphere, however, of my religious heritage: the maternal half which was traceable to the German Palatinate from where, in the late seventeenth century, several of my mother's ancestors migrated to our small valley in eastern Pennsylvania. The paternal half, on the other hand, was predominantly Irish and Roman Catholic—that is, at least, until the early twentieth century when my grandmother scandalized her family by marrying a Campbellite fundamentalist and converting to his faith. These diverse traditions eventually encountered one another when my father's family moved from Connecticut to Pennsylvania during the final years of the Depression.

My father's father had been a successful New England contractor until the economic collapse of the 1930s that nearly bankrupted him.

Then, as if by some favor of Fortune, plans for building a fundamentalist religious college were announced by his church. He applied through a competitive bidding process and was selected as its contractor. Eastern Pennsylvania was chosen as the most desirable location, and a large tract of forested land several miles from our town was purchased for the site. My grandfather bought a small farm adjoining this, which he planned to sell after completing his work and then return to New England; but when the Maranantha Bible Institute (or simply the Institute as it came to be known) project ended three years later, he and my grandmother decided to remain.

My father, however, who was then eighteen and in his final year of high school, did not share his parents' enthusiasm for their new home. Several years before moving with them to Pennsylvania, he had rebelled against his parent's fundamentalism; now, living adjacent to an institution that was a constant reminder of that fact exacerbated the resentment he felt at having his life disrupted. His discontent was softened, however, when he met my mother, who was then twenty-two and taught the senior literature class in which he was enrolled. When he went off to college the following fall, they began seeing each other regularly. Their romance took an impulsive turn with the coming of the war, and they were married the same day he quit school to join the army. In a moment of sober reflection, however, it was mutually agreed that any children would be raised as Lutherans. I was born near the end of the war, and shortly after that we moved into a small frame house that my grandfather had built for us on some land adjoining his farm and the Institute. It was here—and later in my grandfather's large stone farmhouse into which we moved after his death when I was six—that I spent my formative years until moving away permanently after college. Since our property was less than a mile from the Institute (which was also the home of several of my school friends) it was inevitable that I would encounter their religious ideas and rituals.

The entranceway to the Institute was flanked by two imposing stone pillars that stood guard over its access like silent sentinels. Once inside, a narrow road extended straight for nearly a mile through a heavily forested area and then curved sharply to the right, past an open field from which a mammoth wooden tabernacle rose eerily like an architectural apparition. From there the road descended into a clearing where a mass of small wooden cottages, the homes of the students and their families, stood clustered. Further down the hill were a recreation center, two large brick buildings that housed the Institute's educational and administrative spaces, and below these, on a flat plain, a handful of larger faculty residences.

Most of my Saturdays at that time were spent playing at the Institute with the handful of friends who lived there. Occasionally one of them would invite me to spend the night and then accompany the family to church the following morning. During the warm spring and summer months, services were held in the open-sided tabernacle. It had an elevated stage at one end looking out upon endless rows of uncomfortable benches to accommodate the immense congregation, which was much larger than in my own church and incestuously similar in appearance: colorless short-sleeved shirts with loosened ties for the men and unadorned cotton dresses for the women. Only the preacher and his small entourage were distinguished from the crowd by the dark suits they wore.

These worship services were spellbinding affairs, with the preacher pacing the stage like a stalking tiger and modulating his voice synchronously with the rhythms of his body. Sometimes, when just the right emotional lilt had been achieved, an excited parishioner would stand and shout unintelligible phrases, prompting the minister to inform the rapt congregation that God had spoken through the individual as in the Book of Acts: "And they were all filled with the Holy Spirit and began to speak in other tongues, as the Spirit gave them utterance." Near the end of the service, the congregation was encouraged to come forward and "witness" the coming of Jesus into their lives. On more than one occasion, the contagion of the crowd nearly made me join the line trooping toward the stage, but when the time of decision had come and gone, I always found myself riveted as before to the same spot.

This early exposure to two varieties of Christianity with all their ritualistic differences did little to detract from my then unquestioning belief. By the time I was confirmed in the Lutheran church at age twelve, I had even given fleeting consideration to perhaps one day entering the ministry. More importantly, however, it marked a watershed for uncritical faith and acceptance.

Skepticism

Shortly after my confirmation, two events occurred which were to figure prominently in the transformation of my attitude toward God and religion. The first involved a respected local clergyman, Reverend K., then in his early seventies, whose parish church was several towns removed from our own. He had never married and instead had occupied himself with charity, teaching, and scholarship (his written works, for instance, included a diminutive history of his own small Protestant sect and a treatise on St. Augustine). Although we did not attend his church, he was nevertheless acknowledged throughout our valley as a model of the intellectual and pious Christian.

One evening when I was about thirteen, my parents took me to dinner at one of the old country inns that dotted our valley's landscape. The one they chose that night was run by friends of theirs, and it fringed the town in which Reverend K.'s church was located. In the dining room we found ourselves seated next to the table of a distinguished elderly gentleman. He nodded pleasantly to us as we sat down, and my parents discreetly informed me that the man was Reverend K. A short time later after he had finished his dinner, he stopped at our table for a brief conversation since he knew my mother's parents well. To my embarrassment, she proceeded to tell him of my recent confirmation and of the interest I had expressed in the ministry. Before he had an opportunity to reply, she asked him if he still conducted his "famous sessions for young people," addressing those theological issues that adolescents found so perplexing. He smiled graciously and said that he did; then, after extending an invitation to my parents on my behalf, he left us to our dinner. With my appetite gone, I was left with a disquieting image I must have seen once in a movie: that of a timid medieval boy about to be involuntarily apprenticed to a mysterious guildmaster.

Early one evening the following week, my mother drove me the twenty miles to the parsonage where Reverend K. had lived and worked for nearly thirty years. About a dozen boys my own age were there. He introduced me, and I joined them on the library floor as they sat in an arc facing the minister, who reclined in a large leather chair. Next to him was a portable chalkboard, which he used frequently in his efforts to explain difficult concepts. Although he turned out to be a charismatic teacher, two of these sessions in particular stand out in my memory.

The first concerned the Trinity. The subject arose when one of the boys asked the elderly minister why fewer people presently attended church than in the past. Reverend K. began with the conventional explanations—the deterioration of family life and materialism—but then he added one other that seemed mysteriously important, even though none of us comprehended its meaning at the time.

"Most of all, religion is in decline today," he said, "because its symbols have lost their meaning for us. When a society can no longer transform its fears and hopes into meaningful images, it becomes spiritually sick."

We looked at each other, trying to conceal our puzzlement. No one had the courage, however, to interrupt him.

"The Trinity of Father, Son, and Holy Spirit is the most important of all Christian symbols. And" he said, "since we have been created in God's image, we are also a trinity of sorts. However, in our case the three are mind, body, and spirit. And when any one of them is weakened, the entire symbol loses its force. Modern man," he said with a sigh, "no longer believes in the existence of the human spirit. So, if we question our own unity, how can we ever be certain of that vague notion of Father, Son, and Holy Ghost, in whose image we have supposedly been created?"

Reverend K. sat down slowly, his head bowed as if in prayer or contemplation. For a moment he seemed weary, even a little depressed, but after a short silence, he looked up at us and smiled.

"But I am still optimistic," he said firmly. "The Trinity is too powerful a symbol to merely fade away. It is a true image . . . even if St. Paul and the Church Fathers were mistaken and it means something other than Father, Son, and Holy Spirit."

The other session I remember involved his favorite subject: St. Augustine. One evening he was asked whether God ever intervened directly to bring nonbelievers to Christianity. It opened the way for a description of Augustine's conversion and an introduction to the complex problem of evil.

"His story is one of the most remarkable ever written," Reverend K. said with obvious excitement as he retrieved Augustine's *Confessions* from the bookcase. "He was born in a small Roman province in North Africa when the Roman Empire was in decline. From an early age it was apparent that he had a brilliant intellect, but as he grew it also became clear that he had an extreme weakness concerning his own sexual desires. His mother tried to interest him in Christianity, but Augustine thought it much too crude for his intellectual tastes. Finally he was sent to Italy to further his studies, and it was there that he came to recognize the truth contained in the Scriptures. Yet the moral dilemma of his sexual desires still tormented him. One day, as he was sitting beneath a fig tree and wrestling with these passions, Augustine beseeched God to show him the way." Reverend K. opened the *Confessions* and began reading:

All at once I heard the singsong voice of a child in a nearby house—— again and again it repeated the refrain "Take it and read, take it and read." At this I looked up, thinking hard whether there was any kind of game in which children used to chant words like these, but I could not remember hearing them before. I stemmed my flood of tears and stood up, telling myself that this could only be a divine command to open my book of Scripture and read the first passage on which my eyes should fall.

So I hurried back to the place where I had put down the book containing Paul's Epistles. I seized it and opened it and in silence I read the first passage on which my eyes fell: *Not in reveling and drunkenness, not in lust and wantonness, not in quarrels and rivalries. Rather, arm yourselves with the Lord Jesus Christ; spend no more thought on nature and nature's appetites.*[23]

He closed the book and returned it to its place on the shelf. "Augustine recognized that lust is a primary root of evil in this world. It is the sin against which all others can be measured . . . because it is devoid of love. It is an indication of man's fallen state, and all of us share in it because of Adam and Eve's original sin. Augustine's example," he concluded wistfully, "teaches us that only the miracle of divine assistance can help us in overcoming our sinful nature."

That was one of the last sessions I attended, and after that Reverend K. faded from my memory until two years later when I was fifteen. It was then that the secret of his private life became public and, as the story unfolded, Augustine's doctrine of "fallen" man took on a new depth of meaning for me.

For more than twenty years, he had kept a small flat on an obscure back street in a city east of the valley. His prurient passion, it turned out, was a vicarious one for boys around the age of ten. Although he was able to keep his desire repressed near home, he gave it vent monthly during his secretive visits to the city where he would solicit two or three young street boys to engage in erotica with one another while he photographed them. It was reported by several of the boys that Reverend K. preached to them during the ritual something to the effect that "the flesh had to be experienced" before it could be renounced, and that he had been "sent by God" to absorb their sins and to suffer in their place. To symbolize this Christlike sacrifice, at the conclusion of the ordeal, he had them tie his extremities to the bedposts and, once in this modified station of crucifixion, scourge him with thin leather straps which he had brought along for the occasion.

It was inevitable that in the end someone would betray him, and a man who had been one of his early subjects became his Judas in this regard. After being arrested by the city police for an unrelated crime, the man informed them of the minister's activities in an effort to get his own charge reduced. When the case was turned over to the state authorities, they placed the room under surveillance and waited for the right occasion. This came one evening several months later when they broke into the flat just as he was photographing two boys. The next day while searching the parsonage, the police found corroborating evidence in the locked attic. In one corner of the room was a large altar, and behind it hung pictures of Christ surrounded by a throng of adoring children and St. Augustine reclining under a fig tree with a cherubim perched just above his head. On the other walls were compromising photographs of the many children he had solicited and, nailed under each, the thin leather strap used in the rituals of absolution and proxy punishment.

When the local clamor over Reverend K. finally abated many months later, he was quietly committed to a state psychiatric hospital where he spent the remaining years of his life. After becoming a physician myself, I met one of the psychiatrists who was at the facility where Reverend K. had been a patient years before. He related that the elderly minister had been looked upon as something of a prophet by the other patients, although in his final months he became hopelessly delusional. He imagined himself to be the young Augustine and went so far as to keep a bedside Bible opened to that miraculous passage in Paul's Epistles. The psychiatrist did not remember the details of Reverend K.'s death, but he thought it had been a quiet and inoffensive one.

The other episode occurred the year before these revelations about Reverend K. became public. I was fourteen then and still spent most of my Saturdays at the Institute's recreation center playing basketball with my friends. On one of these mornings in early fall, I noticed a girl of eleven or twelve sitting alone in the far bleachers silently watching our play. None of us had seen her come in, and her unexpected presence there almost seemed the product of some conjurer's illusion. I found it nearly impossible to keep from staring at her: she had an exotic face, olive coloring, dark auburn hair, and an impatient figure that seemed poised to unfold like a butterfly from its deceptive chrysalis.

"Who is that?" I asked one of my friends when we broke from play. He looked toward the bleachers.

"Oh that!" he said with a hint of annoyance. "That's Rachael."

"You don't like her?" I asked.

"No," he replied. "And neither does anyone else around here."

"Why?"

"Because she's a snob, and she acts like she knows more than anybody else." He paused to catch his breath. "Her uncle's one of the new teachers here."

"She is pretty, though," I said with conviction.

For the next month Rachael came regularly to watch our Saturday morning play, always sitting quietly by herself off in the distance. I found myself staring at her unconsciously and even rolling the ball toward the place where she sat as an excuse to get nearer. When finally I did manage to see her from several arms' lengths, she looked even more exotic and beautiful than my idealization at a distance had suggested. Then one Saturday she failed to appear and then the Saturday after that, and as the weeks passed, my hopes for her return faded.

On a cold winter morning several months later, I rode my bicycle as usual down the narrow road toward the recreation center. Halfway through the forested area, a small bundled figure became visible in the distance, and as I approached, I recognized it as Rachael walking in my direction. The unexpected sight of her made my throat feel suddenly heavy. But when we came to a stop opposite one another, the sensation faded as she looked up at me and smiled.

"Hello," she said with a friendly air.

I nodded shyly, then stammered, "It's . . . isn't it pretty early to be out . . . alone, I mean?"

"I go out for walks alone all the time," she said, shaking her head.

"And . . . you're not afraid?" I asked.

"No. Why should I be? The Lord watches over all of us." In spite of the unflinching tone, she looked exceptionally fragile standing there bundled up against the winter cold.

"You don't come to watch us play anymore," I said. The inadvertent words poured out spontaneously and the embarrassment showed in the flush of my face.

She shook her head and, as she did, her long hair moved in dark waves over her pink cheeks. "My uncle said I was wasting time. He said I should be praying or reading the Bible instead."

"I was sorry . . . when you stopped coming to watch us." She averted my glance, but there was a faint smile on her lips.

"I go to the youth meeting on Thursday nights," she said suggestively. "My uncle is the pastor. And," she added, "it's open to anyone who wants to hear God's Word."

Before I could respond to her oblique invitation, she had started walking away. As her form waned along the ribbon of road, I felt the sharp pangs of a strange infatuation, which gave me the sensation of being slowly levitated through the cold winter air into a warm current flowing endlessly above it.

That following week I attended my first youth meeting. To make myself less obtrusive, I accompanied my friends from the Institute, who seemed surprised by my request but did not probe my motives too deeply. About twenty children, from ages eight to sixteen, attended regularly, and from my inconspicuous place along the back wall, I could see Rachael clearly as, week after week, she sat in the front row with other girls her own age. Seeing them together merely punctuated the aura of her uniqueness for, next to her, they seemed pale counterfeits.

"Brother" Bob—Rachael's uncle—conducted these Thursday night meetings with the same fervor I had by then become accustomed to. He was accompanied by a tall German expatriate named Karl, who stood mutely to one side of the preacher during the service, looking for all the world more like a soldier than a religious aide. The two of them had met by accident at the end of the war when Bob was stationed in Germany as a military clergyman. He came across the emaciated young man living in the rubble of a bombed building and over the ensuing month, literally nursed him back to health by bringing him daily rations of food and medicine. Once Bob's tour of duty was up, he brought the refugee home with him to America as his assistant. Rachael entered the picture a few years after that; she was the infant daughter of Bob's only sister who had died of complications related to the pregnancy. Since nothing was known about the father, he and Karl took on the task of raising her. This was the official story, in any case. Though rumors occasionally surfaced that Rachael was Bob's—or even Karl's—own child, she bore no resemblance to either of them. Whatever the real truth, the stories only seemed to heighten the mystery surrounding the beautiful little Rachael.

It had been nearly six weeks since I started attending the meetings. The opportunity to talk with her had not arisen because she and her uncle always arrived and left together. Still, I was satisfied merely to be there and to see her—if only from a distance. Then one evening I noticed Rachael waiting alone near the door at the close of the meeting. As I came alongside her, she spoke to me in a whisper.

"Why haven't you talked to me?" Before I could answer, she anxiously added, "My uncle would like to see you."

I followed her silently out of the building and down along the dark path to the cluster of modest faculty houses about a quarter of a mile away. When we entered her living room, Karl and Bob were sitting there in stiff chairs facing the doorway. Her uncle got up and welcomed me with a faint smile, while Karl remained seated and mute. As Bob motioned me to the sofa opposite them, Rachael crossed over and sat on the floor next to her uncle's chair.

"Do you enjoy our meetings?" he asked after a long silence.

"Yes," I responded.

"I believe you belong to one of those old established churches in town."

I nodded, then looked toward Rachael who was staring at the floor. That he knew anything at all about me made me vaguely uncomfortable. And the long pause that followed merely sustained that sensation.

"Why then do you come to *our* meetings?" he said with sudden brusqueness, his original smile turning into a grimace.

The severity of his tone startled me, and I felt the skin of my palms and face moisten. When I tried to fashion a response, the poorly formed words lodged in my dry throat.

"I believe *I* know the answer," he responded without waiting for me to speak. He looked down at his niece. "Rachael told me that she had invited you to our meetings. At first, I didn't think anything of it—that is, until I noticed you staring at her week after week. And," he added," until she began mentioning 'that new boy' just a little too often."

My greatest desire at that moment was to look at Rachael, but my fear of being detected prevented it. Still, there was some consolation in knowing that she thought of me at all. When I managed the courage to look in his direction again, I noticed that he was gazing down at her.

"Rachael is a very special child. . . . God has given her the gifts of prophecy and healing." He did not elaborate on this, but his voice sounded softer and less threatening. "She has dedicated herself to His work, and no temptation will be allowed to lead her astray."

His last words recalled Reverend K.'s portrait of Augustine and the theme of mankind's struggle in the face of worldly seductions. Yet I could not fathom its analogy to the innocent situation involving Rachael and me.

"I have nothing against you, but I must protect Rachael—just as, in the Bible, Laban protected his Rachel."

For the first time since his rebuke had started, he smiled noticeably in my direction and then gently stroked his niece's hair. Then there was a long silence. Finally, he got up from his chair and walked me to the door while Rachael remained seated on the floor.

"I'm sure your church has its own youth meetings," he said while he motioned to his silent assistant. "It's late, Karl. Please drive the boy home."

For months after that I avoided the Institute, making a series of feeble excuses to my friends about staying away. The memory of my inquisition was too much alive and painful; even the thought of seeing Rachael again could not blot it out. Inevitably, however, the sting gradually became less piercing, and after a four-month absence, I returned to the Institute and my friends.

On an early Saturday in spring a few weeks after that, I turned as usual onto the long stretch of road that led into the Institute. Halfway ahead the figure of a small girl walking with her back toward me came suddenly into view. Then, just as suddenly, it vanished into the dense forest on the left. I rode to the place where she had disappeared and pulled my bicycle into the foliage. Although I had only glimpsed her, there was little doubt that the figure had been Rachael's and that she had not seen my approach. For an instant the unpleasant image of her uncle flashed before me, then faded almost as rapidly. Soon I found myself under the canopy of tall trees close to the spot where she had turned in. Although I had never explored the forest, I knew from my friends' stories that it was bordered by the Institute on one side and, about a mile distant, on the other by a wide lake rimmed with stone hills which were said to contain a network of shallow caverns.

A dozen yards from my entry point, I came across an old Indian path that plumbed the woods and uncoiled in the general direction of the lake. Although I could neither see nor hear her, I knew that Rachael was somewhere up ahead. The warm morning light penetrated the forest cover, bathing its interior with a soft glow, and every now and then I came across snapped branches or disturbed undergrowth indicating someone else's presence there before me. I walked as quietly as possible, which made the path seem endless, but after nearly an hour, the trees finally thinned and directly ahead I saw the lake reflected in the blue sunlight; to the right of it was a sheer rocky precipice on the face of which were the numerous small perforations of caverns. Turning from the path toward the granite butte, I became aware of a faint sound coming from one of the ground-level caves. Its entranceway was camouflaged by several large bushes, and by settling quietly behind these, I was able to see clearly into the interior without being seen in turn.

The cave's portico was a narrow alcove that billowed upward like the nave of a medieval church. A yellow glow, probably originating from a breach in the vaulted ceiling, illuminated the interior and its bizarre furnishings: a small wooden table with three mismatched chairs arranged around it, and crates, plates and pots, candles, and various other oddities; even several indistinct pictures hung from the rough stone walls. Through this impoverished maze—which must have taken months of small convoys to assemble—Rachael talked to herself and to three floppy dolls seated around the table.

"Eat all of your lunch, Dorothy," she lectured to the largest doll. "See that! Your brother and sister are watching, and you must be a good example to them."

Moving to the male doll, she declared, "John, you can't go out until . . ." She looked back at Dorothy. "See! Your sister is eating now."

After a few moments she lifted the two dolls from their chairs and placed them near the caves' narrow entrance. She waved to them as if they were going out to play, and then she returned to the table, picked up the smallest doll, and sat down with it cradled in her lap.

"They are very naughty!" She gently rocked the female infant and, after several minutes, said, "You must take a nap before your father gets home." She got up, laid the doll in a small crate, and covered it with a tattered pink towel.

From my hiding place in the shadow of the cave's entrance, I could see her distinctly as she hummed and happily busied herself with the tasks of her private fantasy world. Although I desperately wanted to make my presence known, I sensed that any interruption of her complex illusion would be terribly cruel. At last I decided to steal away, but as I backed from my hiding place, Rachael appeared, walked out into the morning sunlight, and stood in the doorway of the cave.

"Are you there?" she whispered.

I crouched down, thinking she had seen me, but instead she was looking skyward where a solitary pair of hawks were circling above the far shore. Then she clasped her hands over her small breasts in a gesture of supplication.

"Thank you for giving me this secret place." She looked down at the dolls propped in the doorway. "And for them . . . and for my uncle . . . and for Karl . . . and for my mother who is with you in heaven . . . and for the other children at the Institute . . . and," she concluded, "for that quiet boy who paid attention to me."

A small flock of noisy waterfowl swept down on their approach to the lake. They landed on the water with a flourish, but Rachael did not seem to hear the commotion. Instead, she bent down onto her knees and turned her gaze skyward toward the symbolic realm of heaven.

"I am frightened, God," she said slowly with a tone of genuine anguish. "When I am inside my house I can't seem to feel you near." There was a pause. "It makes me feel guilty to be so happy then." For many minutes after that, I saw only the silent movement of her lips; finally she got up, lifted the two dolls propped near the entranceway, and turned to go inside.

"My uncle said that happiness can be a sin and that the worst punishment of all is when you turn away from someone . . ." Her voice trailed off into inaudibility. As she disappeared into the cave's interior, I got up quietly from my hiding place and retreated into the forest.

I saw Rachael only once more after that: she was walking near the spot where I had seen her vanish into the woods that day. As I passed on my bicycle, she waved, but owing to my embarrassment at the theft of her secret, I could not bring myself to stop. The following autumn she, her uncle, and Karl left the Institute permanently and settled somewhere in the Midwest.

A few years later the lake and its tributary were dammed up to supply water to the surrounding counties. The expanding reservoir submerged more than half the forest bordering the Institute—including Rachel's cave. I am certain that her sanctuary lies there today, peacefully preserved. More than Rachael's shrine, however, it is also a symbolic sepulcher to God's memory. For it was within that sanctuary, where she was happiest, that Rachael discovered God's absence: the same entombed absence with which Nietzsche concluded the story of his madman over a century ago:

> It has been related further that on that same day the madman entered diverse churches and there sang his *requiem aeternam deo*. Led out and called to account, he is said to have replied each time, "What are these churches now if they are not the tombs and sepulchers of God?"[24]

SEVEN

NEAR THE SUMMIT OF THE SEVEN STOREY MOUNTAIN

THE PROBLEM OF free will, like Kant's other two metaphysical postulates (the soul's immortality and God's existence), is destined to lie forever beyond man's reach. But while there may be no definite *solution*, there is at least an *answer*: admit that one's freedom may be a delusion, but postulate it nevertheless; or, more radically still, begin with the primal self as the existentialists have done and assert that freedom is the one human constant that determines what we are and what we will become. Reconciling consciousness of ourselves as free agents with our everyday experiences thus brings us face-to-face with the irreducible question of *human nature* itself.

Modern psychiatry and psychology are adrift with theories about human nature. But there was one individual long ago who anticipated many of their ideas. It was as a college freshman that I first encountered him.

The Professor and the Poet

Except for his shorter stature and larger forehead, Professor O. bore a striking resemblance to the actor Richard Burton. Like this famous counterpart, his passion was for the dramatic arts, which formed part of the English curriculum. As one of the junior faculty, however, he was also expected to teach his share of introductory classes. Of these, the most important was the required freshman course in Western

Literature. By a stroke of good fortune, I found myself assigned to his class.

From the first, the professor made his literary preferences clear to all of us: Shakespeare occupied the position of preeminence, followed by Dante, and then Milton. Nevertheless, he spent more time on Dante's *Divine Comedy* than any author's single work. Although I did not appreciate its worth at the time, Professor O. made the tour through Dante's universe memorable enough for me to still remember much of it.

"Imagine yourself in Dante's Italy of the late Middle Ages," he began. "You will find an atmosphere dominated by the Church. As you might expect then, Dante's education was largely theological. But since he came from a genteel family, it also included philosophy and the idealized poetry of the day. It was through this latter influence that he created literature's most celebrated *donna angelicata*. I am referring, of course," he said reverently, "to the ethereal Beatrice."

Only a few of us had ever heard of Beatrice, and only one raised her hand when he asked if anyone had read Dante's classic in its entirety. "Excellent," he said with a wry smile. "I see then that only one of you will require the extra work needed to erase the faulty impressions implanted by previous teachers."

Benign as this sarcasm was, it nevertheless expressed his genuine sentiment that works as ethereal as Shakespeare's or Dante's had no place in a freshman introductory course. They required maturity and a catalogue of lived experience, he said on more than one occasion, before they could be appreciated. He feared that encountering them prematurely might bias the student against their "strangeness" and discourage their future reading. There was indeed truth in this conviction.

After some comments about the author's personal life, Professor O. went on to discuss the various interpretations applied by critics to Dante's imaginary journey through Hell, Purgatory, and Paradise: the moral (as an instructive story about the consequences of various behaviors); the literal (as an autobiography of journeys and adventures); and the allegorical (as a mystical Christian vision of God's grand design for the universe). To these he added a fourth of his own.

"Most of all," he said, "I view Dante's work as a treatise on *human nature*—perhaps the most thoughtful one ever written—and as a tribute to the transforming power of love symbolized, of course, by Beatrice. But I am getting ahead of myself. Let us begin with his opening line— and perhaps literature's most famous statement of a midlife crisis." He read from the text:

> Midway in the journey of our life I found myself in a dark wood, for the straight way was lost.

"Dante cannot remember how he happened to be there," the professor continued, "because in his words: 'I was so full of sleep at the moment I left the true way.' Searching for an exit, he comes to a mountain whose summit is suffused with light. But his path is blocked by three fearsome beasts. As he retreats to avoid their onslaught, the ghost of the Roman poet Virgil (representing human reason) appears and tells Dante that he has been sent by Beatrice (divine love) to guide him from the valley."

The professor rearranged the books and papers on his desk. "The route she has chosen for Dante, however, is a circuitous one: instead of a direct path out of the valley, he and his guide will descend into Hell; then climb the terraces of Purgatory; and finally, journey upwards through the circles of Heaven. Next time," he said as the hour came to a close, "we will accompany our two travelers as they begin."[25]

Over the ensuing weeks Professor O. guided us through Dante's three realms. Although most of the time was devoted to his journey through Hell (with its inventive tortures), it was his ascent of Purgatory which held a special and mysterious relevance for me.

Purgatory

"When Lucifer was cast from Heaven," the professor began his lecture on Dante's second canticle, "the impact brought him to rest near the earth's center and created Hell in the process. But the fall also pushed up a tall mountain—Mount Purgatory—on the earth's surface opposite the impact. There, to make up for the loss of his favorite angel, God created Adam and Eve and placed them in a garden near its summit. Unfortunately, this second creation turned out to be even more troublesome than the first.

"But God did not give up on mankind as he had on Lucifer," he continued. "Through Purgatory he provided him a final opportunity for salvation. First, he had to purify himself by ascending the mountain; then, if successful, he was admitted to the lost Eden at its summit. From there, Paradise was but a step away."

Dante's conception of Purgatory was consistent with the Christian theology of his day. Within its moral "geography" (midway between Hell and Heaven), man's lesser transgressions were punished. Here the contrite sinner could be made worthy of ransoming a second moment in mankind's lost earthly paradise before finally ascending to Heaven. Purgatory thus represented Dante's symbolic journey through the world of moral philosophy, one which was guided primarily by human reason in the person of the dead poet Virgil.

"Reason, however, will be able to take Dante only so far," Professor O. warned. "Virgil will disappear from the drama after he has led our hero through Purgatory's seven terraces; thereafter Beatrice, the symbol of divine love, will serve as his guide."

The terraces, or storeys,[26] to which the professor referred were the seven ascending steppes of Mount Purgatory, each corresponding to one of the "deadly sins" which were sequentially purged there. Unlike Hell, where punishment was the aim, Purgatory was a school of moral instruction where the inhabitants engaged hopefully in their labors. And whereas Dante was only an observer in Hell, in

Purgatory he became an active participant in its purifying rituals. Stripped of its embroidery, his seven-storey climb had a simple configuration:

1) On the lowest terrace were the *proud*, who did penance under a heavy load of stone in order to learn humility;

2) Next came the *envious*, who had their eyelids sutured shut to make them dependent upon each other for support;

3) After this were the *angry*, who chanted in unison the Agnus Dei in order to teach themselves meekness;

4) Then came the *slothful*, constantly in motion, in order that "zeal in doing well [might] renew grace";

5) Next were the *avaricious*, who lay prostrate, staring at the earth— because in life their gaze was "fixed upon earthly things"—as a lesson in liberality;

6) Then came the *gluttonous*, emaciated by hunger and thirst, who were kept in constant sight of a stream and the fruit-laden trees on its banks, as a lesson in temperance; and

7) On the last terrace stood the *lustful*, who were purified of their excesses in a wall of flame.

"These seven sins (and their corresponding virtues) sum up perfectly the condition of mankind," he remarked. "At the same time, he has given us the means to understanding and overcoming these human imperfections. That key is love, as we will see when we meet Beatrice in the earthly paradise at the summit of Mount Purgatory."

Although I was unaware of it then, the readings that followed would have several strange, personal parallels. They were foreshadowed in a few brief passages which the professor took up in his next lecture.

"After passing through the flames of the seventh terrace," he began, "Dante and Virgil find themselves on the steps leading to the garden.

With night approaching, they stop there to sleep, and near daybreak Dante has a prophetic dream." The professor read from the text:

I seemed to see in a dream a lady young and beautiful going through a meadow gathering flowers and, singing, she was saying, "Whoso asks my name, let him know that I am Leah, and I go moving my fair hands around to make myself a garland. To please me of the glass I adorn me here, but my sister Rachel never leaves her mirror and sits all day long. She is fair to behold her eyes, as I am to deck me with my hands: *She with seeing I with doing am satisfied.*

Reading this passage the night before class had awakened a brief reminiscence of my own Rachael, but when Professor O. explained its symbolism, it took on a new significance. These two biblical sisters were popular medieval symbols of the active (Leah) and contemplative (Rachel) life—the former roaming the fields and picking flowers and the latter peering into her soul as mirrored through her eyes.[27]

Leah would have her counterpart in Dante's drama as Matelda, the beautiful lady of the garden, while Rachel would portend the appearance of Beatrice. In Dante's symbolic world, Leah and Matelda were thus the ideals of earthly love, while Rachel and Beatrice were their spiritual counterparts.

Professor O. completed his synopsis: After awakening, Dante began exploring the "divine forest" that lay before him. Soon he came upon a narrow stream. On its opposite bank he saw a beautiful lady (Matelda), singing to herself and culling flowers from a nearby meadow. She described how God had given mankind this terrestrial paradise as a place of eternal peace, but that through sinfulness he had exchanged "honest joy and sweet sport for tears and toil." The stream separating them, she explained, was one of two that fed the garden. Their waters had special powers since they originated from a holy spring near the mountain's summit: one, called Lethe, removed all memory of sin, while the other,

Eunoe, restored memories of past good deeds. It was her task to wash those who had been purged on the terraces below in their waters in preparation for the final ascent into Paradise.

As Matelda (Leah) led him along the stream's bank, a dazzling processional suddenly appeared. In it were a host of symbolic figures drawn from the Bible with a triumphal chariot at its center. When the processional came to a stop, the participants invoked the climactic appearance of Beatrice—the symbolic counterpart of Rachel in his dream.

Dante immediately recognized Beatrice as his former earthly love whom death had prematurely claimed. She chided him before the assembly for being unfaithful to her memory and pursuing the path of illusory goods. The only way to save him, she explained, was to arrange a journey of self-discovery through Hell and then Purgatory. He was now ready, she declared, to visit the blessed in Paradise with her as guide.

Rita's Earthly Paradise

When Professor O.'s "Introduction to Western Literature" came to a close, I found to my astonishment that I had enjoyed it even more than my science courses. The following year I managed to enroll in another of his classes—this time a theatre arts elective. In some respects, this second encounter with the humanities was even more satisfying than the first, and I found myself beginning to question my commitment to science as a career. I decided, however, to make another effort at rekindling my interest by registering for a special summer research program that was being offered by the college. In that way, I thought I could make a more objective assessment of my interests before the start of the fall semester. As it turned out, that experience only complicated matters more. In the end, a decision was made more by default than reason.

That summer I rented a small apartment a short distance from the college's science complex. (I had no car and depended upon walking or bicycling to get where I needed to go.) One morning early in the session, I passed Professor O. on my way to the laboratory. He seemed pleased to see me, and we stopped to talk.

"It occurs to me," he said after the greetings were over, "that you might be interested in coming out to the Playhouse in the evening. You could help with some of our productions—after all, you know the rudiments of theatre after taking my course this spring—which, I might add, you did damned well in." With good-natured sarcasm, he inserted, "For a scientist, that is."

"I just *cannot* understand the allure that science has for so many of you nowadays," he continued. "There *are* other ways of getting at the truth, you know. Or is there something more profound about it that I am overlooking?"

His question seemed directly aimed at my own growing conflict over science and the arts. At that moment, however, I did not want to involve myself in a discussion of it, so I answered, "I'm afraid I don't know."

"Nor do I," he said with a smile. "In any event, come out and join us—even if it's just for the fun of it." I thanked him and promised to consider it.

The following afternoon I bicycled into the deserted countryside and followed the directions he had given me. The summer heat had not yet reached its zenith, and scattered wildflowers still bloomed by the roadside. Although the road tracked through undulating terrain, the five-mile ride was an agreeable one. Soon a large sign appeared, marking the entrance to the theatre. The "Playhouse," as it was simply named, was easily visible from the roadway. It had been converted from an old barn and was painted a deep crimson in keeping with its original color. To add a personal touch, the professor had colored the window casements and trim sapphire and green, giving it the appearance of a bright chalet stuck in the middle of nowhere. Behind the Playhouse was a large, un-mowed field which fanned out in a semicircle, and around its circumference was a dense wood. In the far left corner of the meadow, the loop of a narrow stream could be seen as it arced out of the forest and then returned again.

Half a dozen cars were parked in the theatre's front lot, and an old pickup truck laden with planks and painted canvases was backed up to the open entrance. From there I could see the theatre's interior perfectly. It had a rustic, cathedral-like quality due to its arched ceiling, which was crisscrossed by long, thin beams from which hung several types of theatre lights. Its focal point, however, was a round central stage which took up nearly half of the theatre's floor space. There were about a dozen people there, and Professor O. stood in the center directing their activities. I went unnoticed for several minutes until he inadvertently looked in my direction and then motioned me to come ahead.

Many of those milling about were college students I knew—by name or face primarily—from school productions. They formed the core of the professor's small troupe, which also included two "professional" actors from New York City who had been hired on as summer headliners. Since the opening of his summer stock theatre five years before, these out-of-towners had become a staple of Professor O's productions. (Most of them were obscure actors who were paid very little, but that was of secondary importance compared to the experience they gained.) After some introductions, the professor asked me to help several of the others assemble the props that were to be used in the opening night performance scheduled for the following weekend. The two students assigned the job had nearly finished by that time, however, and with nothing further to do, I walked outside to look around.

Something drew me to the meadow behind the Playhouse that I had glimpsed from the road. But as I got to the edge of the building and was about to turn in that direction, I was held there by a fascinating sight. In the meadow near the stream was an attractive young woman in a white flowing dress who seemed to be singing to herself as she bent to pick from the clumps of wildflowers that grew near the water's edge. Before the scene could fully impress itself on me, however, its tranquility was broken by Professor O., who whisked around the corner of the building.

"Where in God's name is she?" he mumbled to himself—then to me, as if I would know to whom he was referring. Scanning the meadow and seeing her there, he called out, "Rita! We are waiting to rehearse your lines." Then with more composure, he said, "Please hurry, dear."

His call startled the young woman, for she quickly wrapped her flowers in a scarf and hastened toward us. As we stood watching, the professor could not conceal his annoyance. He grumbled loudly enough for me to hear: "Goddamned New York actors—they seem to think that this is a paid vacation." But when she got close enough to touch, his ethos suddenly changed. "Rita," he purred, "we were worried about you." Then, looking at her white dress, his sense of realism returned. "I hope you haven't gotten stains on your costume."

"I'm sorry," she said, shaking her head, "but I only now discovered that little brook in the corner of the meadow." She turned and looked in its direction. "There must be twenty different types of wildflowers growing there." As she opened up her white scarf to show us, their multicolored petals cascaded against the silken background. She offered one to the professor and then to me.

"They are beautiful," he agreed, "but we must go in—the others are waiting." He turned to me. "Would you mind putting these in water for Rita?" Without waiting for a reply, he took the flowers from her, handed them to me, and abruptly escorted her inside.

That was my first encounter with Rita. Over the ensuing weeks I would learn much more about her. But until then I knew only what I heard and what I could observe for myself—that she was twenty-five, a native New Yorker, and an aspiring actress with an exquisitely expressive face and bright oval eyes. She had been accompanied for the summer by a fellow New York actor, a tall black man in his early forties, whose stage name was simply "Jason." Since he had several minor off-Broadway successes to his credit, the professor gave him top billing that summer over Rita. To those of us who watched the rehearsals and the finished productions, however, it was apparent that her talent, though unpolished, was more profound than his. Jason seemed to sense this, too, because his public treatment of her was often dismissive—although most of us suspected that privately they were lovers. The net effect was that it kept most of us at a distance from them while at the same time compelling us to watch discretely for any subtle signs of intimacy. In the end I would know the truth, while the others would be left with only their intuitions.

Rita kept to herself as much as possible. When not rehearsing she seemed to prefer the meadow and forest, where the wildflowers were still in bloom, to the company of others. Because I was the most expendable member of the company, the professor assigned me the task of retrieving her whenever she was needed for rehearsals. Usually it was sufficient for me to stand at the rear of the Playhouse and call out; although sometimes, when she strayed into the neighboring woods, I would have to wander out to the tree line and call from there. After several minutes she inevitably appeared, and then we would return together to the Playhouse. For the first week these were quiet walks, but with the growing predictability of my appearances, she began to shed her reserve.

One day Rita broke the silence as she walked beside me carrying an especially large collection of flowers. "In case you're wondering, I press these each night after rehearsal. I have filled nearly two books, and these should get me started on a third," she said.

"What do you know about your flowers?" I asked with scientific curiosity.

She shook her head. "What does one need to know about them . . . except that they are beautiful?"

"I guess that is enough." We reached the back wall of the Playhouse and stopped there for a moment before going inside.

"When I was a little girl, I remember finding some old books in my grandmother's attic that were full of pressed flowers. After all those years they still had their delicate shapes—even some of their original color." She sighed. "What stories those flowers might have told if only they had voices!"

I wanted to tell her that I too had once discovered something in my grandparents' attic. It was a box of dusty old shoes, and I remembered making up stories about the imaginary roads they had walked along. But the comparison with wildflowers made a story about shoes seem too irreverent to mention.

"You may have these," she said, handing me her bouquet. "That is, if you promise to press them. Then, in twenty or thirty years, you can hide the books in a corner of your own attic for your children's children."

Over the following weeks Rita's history took form through these little exchanges as we walked to and from the meadow. She had been born in a small town in upstate New York where three generations of her family had lived. Her mother taught elementary school and her father worked at assorted construction jobs. When she was three they moved to New York City, where a flood of building projects promised her father steady employment. A short time later, however, he contracted a rare illness—some type of leukemia, Rita thought—and was dead within three months. Through his life insurance and her mother's small income they managed to live modestly, however. Her mother never remarried, and Rita saw her infrequently now.

It was plain from her descriptions that she and her mother shared similar temperaments: both were shy and introverted, although Rita considered herself the more afflicted of the two. To help overcome this, she took up high school dramatics and, finding that she had talent and enjoyed it, continued it in college. Following graduation she decided to try it as a career. At first the parts were scarce, but with her ability and persistence, the offers gradually multiplied and she found herself working more often than not. Her summers, however, were reserved for out-of-the-way stock companies where she could experiment with new roles and get a respite from city life.

One day as we walked back from the meadow together, I noticed that she was particularly quiet. Her large oval eyes appeared misty and sad.

"Is something the matter?" I asked.

"I found only these today." She showed me a half-dozen anemic flowers that had endured the midsummer heat.

"The wildflower season is apparently near its end," I said.

"Then I'm glad that I preserved as many of them as I did." She sighed. "It doesn't matter though. Fate never reveals her plans in advance."

"Fate?" I could not conceal the hint of skepticism in my voice.

"You don't believe in it?"

"I don't know . . ."

She paused. "I have experienced too many coincidences not to believe in its possibility."

My personal experiences to that time had convinced me that Fate—and its religious equivalent, "God's Will"—was nothing more than a convenient excuse for relieving one of personal responsibility. However, her conviction seemed so genuine that I found myself wanting to believe as she did, while at the same time harboring the strange sense that her words were prologue to something more.

"Haven't you wondered, for instance," she said, "whether our being here together at this moment might not have something to do with Fate?"

"I . . . I'm not sure."

What followed was unprompted and sequenceless. We briefly brushed against each other, and our glances met. Everything else around us seemed momentarily unreal—except for the image of inevitability that we saw reflected in each other's look. That night after rehearsal was over, I waited for Rita in the shadows near the highway entrance. On the drive back to town, we sat quietly until she stopped the car in front of her apartment. After she turned the engine and lights off, we sat there in the dark for a few minutes more.

"Does this make you uncomfortable?" Rita finally asked.

"No . . . at least I don't think so."

"Are you sure?"

"Well, I suppose there is something I would like to ask." She turned in the seat to face me. "It's about you and . . . Jason."

"Jason?" She paused for a few moments. "You mean you thought that . . ." She began to laugh softly.

"I didn't think it was funny!"

"Don't you see," she said, "Jason is, well . . . my decoy . . . my protector. If people think he is more than that, they aren't very likely to bother me, are they?"

"I suppose not."

"Jason is only a friend." She touched my hand.

There was a certain dreamlike quality to the weeks that followed, as if they had been fused onto a surrealist's canvas. But though the flow of time and events seemed to merge into a continuum, there were occasions when the images took on more distinctness as the words on a page do when one concentrates on the whiteness between them. The most vivid of these occurred one afternoon toward the end of summer. Rita had wandered off as usual behind the Playhouse. A few minutes later I slipped away to join her. She was waiting near the bank of the small stream where it looped briefly across the meadow's edge.

"I want to show you something," she said eagerly.

Rita led me into the forest along the bank of the brook. Soon the stream narrowed, and at a place where several large rocks projected above its surface, we crossed over to the other side. Here she stopped and faced me.

"Close your eyes," she said.

"Close my eyes . . . why?"

"Please do as I say," she entreated.

"Oh, all right." She took her white silk scarf from around her waist and tied it around the upper part of my face as a blindfold.

"Now, take my arm," she commanded.

She took my hand and guided it there. Then she began leading me slowly along the irregular path. It was a bizarre sensation to be without sight in an unfamiliar place. Even her careful navigation could not prevent me from stumbling every now and then on the branches and rocks that had collected along the way.

"Why are we doing this?" I asked after we had walked for some time.

"Because I want to surprise you."

"I thought that it was to be sure that I couldn't find this place—wherever it is you are taking me—without your help."

She laughed as she squeezed my hand. "Perhaps that too. But only unconsciously." After a few more minutes, we stopped. "We're here," she said, removing the scarf while I rubbed my eyes and blinked several times to adjust to the light. "What do you think of it?"

The place that Rita had brought me to was a small circular clearing deep in the woods from which I could glimpse neither the meadow nor the stream. Later she told me that she had come upon it while searching for the last of the summer wildflowers, which covered the ground here in spite of the lateness of the season. The curious aura of the place, however, had kept her from picking any of them. There was indeed something out of the ordinary about this small tract of forest that Rita had accidentally discovered. It bore little resemblance to the woods that nearly hid it from view.

Half of its perimeter was ringed by medium-sized trees unlike any others in the forest. They appeared to be equally spaced, mirror images of one another, and each looked as if it had been chosen with care and placed there by design. Even the lines of bark seemed to be interchangeable from one tree to the next. Enclosing the other half of the perimeter was a semicircular rock ledge about eight feet high. The stones comprising it were large squares that seemed perfectly fitted, and near the center of the arc, a small spring bubbled forth through the rock about a foot from the ground. Its waters cut a narrow trench along the base in both directions as if two miniature streams—exact duplicates flowing opposite one another—had been created by the spring. Then, at the two concluding edges of wall, the waters disappeared abruptly, apparently swallowed up by some natural drainage system beneath the ledge. The enclosure's interior was much simpler, but no less symmetrical. The ground there was perfectly flat and covered by a dense layer of purple-hued forest grass that gave it the appearance of a soft carpet. The only other object within the clearing was an immense smooth stone at its very center that resembled the edge of a large egg buried halfway into the earth with a portion of one pole protruding.

"What do you think of my discovery?" Rita asked excitedly.

"I . . . I don't know what to say. I've never seen anything quite like it." She led me to the center of the clearing where we sat together on the granite egg.

"It looks too orderly to be a work of nature," she mused. "But on the other hand, it can't be a human creation."

In spite of its fascination, something about the enclosure made me uncomfortable. Its grating symmetry compared with the surrounding forest created an uneasy feeling within. "Maybe it's the work of the little people—you know, elves or leprechauns," I said in an effort to disarm the sensation.

Instead of responding, Rita stared at the stone ledge and the fountain at its center. Then, just as I was about to speak again, she said, "There is something vaguely familiar about this place. It's almost as if I have been here before. I know that is impossible, but I feel it nevertheless."

"Perhaps you saw a picture or read a story that reminded you of it. Psychologists say that sort of thing happens all the time."

"I suppose you're right."

Rita seemed slightly dejected by my attempt to explain it away scientifically. Her comments, however, had opened up my own set of associations which, after a time, became too strongly coincidental to keep private.

"Now that I think of it, this place reminds me of something too." Rita's face brightened a little. "Do you remember reading Dante in college?" I asked.

"Yes. I can't say that I really enjoyed him though."

"Do you recall the earthly paradise near the summit of Purgatory?"

"Only faintly, I'm afraid. Wasn't that supposed to represent the Garden of Eden?"

I nodded. "And Dante had a dream while he was waiting to enter it: a vision of Rachel and her sister—what was her name?—oh yes, Leah. And when he awoke, he met Matelda, the beautiful lady who tended the garden and eventually delivered Dante to Beatrice."

For some reason the details of Dante's *Purgatory* bubbled up with remarkable vividness. I told Rita what I remembered: the seven sins that were purged in preparation for entrance into the garden; Dante's dream about Rachel and Leah and its symbolism; Matelda, the symbol of earthly love, whom Dante had first encountered singing to herself and picking flowers in a meadow near a stream—as I had seen Rita doing that first day behind the Playhouse; the two rivers, Lethe and Eunoe, originating in a sacred spring at Purgatory's summit—as the two miniature streams here flowed from a small fountain along the base of Rita's wall; and Beatrice, the symbol of spiritual love.

"So I remind you of Leah . . . and Matelda, was it?"

"Yes," I replied. "But it never occurred to me until this moment."

"But why not Beatrice—and Rachel? Don't misunderstand me," she added. "I am honored by the comparison with Leah and Matelda. But Beatrice was Dante's leading character. Why not her instead of Matelda? Was it the meadow and the flowers?"

"I suppose so. In any case, Beatrice struck me as too spiritual to be real. Matelda, on the other hand, was . . ."

"Was worldly?"

"Yes. I could never imagine Beatrice making love; it would seem almost sacrilegious . . ."

"Then you have a lot to learn about women," she said, smiling. "There is some of Matelda inside all of us, to be sure—but Beatrice is there too."

Her comments brought back the memory of my own Rachael who, like her namesake and Dante's Beatrice, had been groomed for otherworldliness. I wondered whether she was doomed to sainthood like them or whether the Matelda-Leah inside of her had been freed.

"What are you thinking?" Rita asked.

"I was wondering what it would be like to make love in this soft grass," I said half-jokingly.

"It wouldn't work—I feel too much like Beatrice right now." She was quiet for a time and then said abruptly, "We should get back to the Playhouse. Suddenly this place looks very ordinary to me."

"Did I say something that offended you?"

"No. I just need some time to think," she said. We walked back to the Playhouse in silence.

For the next few days, as if by some unspoken covenant, we did not see each other. Then several more elapsed before our relationship began reviving. But though things seemed to go on much as before, it was clear that something had irrevocably altered in Rita since that day in the forest. A few weeks after that the Playhouse closed, and we spent our last day together. In the morning she would depart for New York and I would return home for a week before the start of the fall classes.

"What will you do now that summer is over?" Rita asked as we lay quietly in bed staring at the fragments of moonlight refracted upon the ceiling.

"I'm not sure. School starts again in a week—that doesn't leave time for much of anything."

As I held her hand, the pulsations transmitted from her heart to my fingers were easily discernible. Her breathing was regularly spaced between every eighth to tenth beat. I noticed that my own pulse and heart rate had synchronized with hers as if through some biological bond of sympathy.

"I'm sorry about the last few weeks," she said after a long silence. "I haven't been myself, and I owe you an explanation."

"You don't have to explain," I answered.

"But I do—and I want to."

"If you think you must," I said, trying to disguise my curiosity.

"When I came across that place in the woods," she began, "it was as if I had found a miniature paradise waiting there just for me. I even felt as if Fate had singled me out for its discovery. But then when I took you there, that all changed somehow with your talk of Dante and Purgatory. The image I had seemed to dissolve right in front of me. Please don't misunderstand," she quickly added. "I'm not blaming you. In fact, I am grateful for what you made me see—and understand."

"I never meant to ruin it for you," I said

She turned onto her side and faced me. "I know you didn't."

"But how could you possibly be grateful if I . . . ?" She placed her fingers on my lips.

"I didn't like Dante when he was forced on me in college," she continued. "He seemed to be just another irrelevant dead author. But when you pointed out the analogies between his earthly paradise near Purgatory's summit and mine beyond the meadow—and when you said that I reminded you of Leah and of Dante's Matelda—I knew in my heart that the imagery was accurate. *Depressingly* accurate."

"But why should that make you feel depressed?"

"Because I suddenly realized that I hadn't earned my admission. I knew it when you described Dante's descent into Hell and then his climb up Purgatory . . . and all the sins that had to be purged along the way before he was allowed to enter the garden. I suppose it depressed me to realize how much more perfecting there was for me to do before I would be worthy of recovering any lost paradise."

"But at least you got a glimpse of it—or at least something resembling it," I said encouragingly.

"Yes," she responded, resting her head upon my shoulder. "I think that somewhere inside each of us is this same vague sense of having lost something precious—and more perfect than this everyday world."

"I think I understand," I said.

There seemed to be little more to say after that, and we lay there quietly until morning came a short time later. I helped Rita load her things into the car for the trip home, and then we drove to the local diner to wait for Jason. After he arrived, Rita and I wandered off for a few last minutes together, and afterward I watched her drive off with Jason following behind. I knew it would be the last time I would see her. As with Rachael before her, this symbolic Leah too had gone. All that remained were their immutable images as *anima*—and each reflected a facet of death: for Rachael, the death of God; for Rita, the death of a dream.

That afternoon, before leaving for home, I rode out to the deserted Playhouse and walked back through the meadow and along the stream to the place Rita had discovered. I sat on the egg-shaped stone in the center of the clearing and surveyed her paradise, which now appeared quite ordinary: the trees seemed slightly bent, and the blocks of the stone wall looked more random than I had remembered them. By next summer, I knew that everything here would be hidden within the camouflage of the surrounding forest. And it occurred to me that, but for Rita, it had always been that way.

EIGHT

LIFE IS THAT WHICH MEN CALL DEATH— AND VICE VERSA

"Whence this pleasing hope
This longing after immortality?
Eternity! thou pleasing, dreadful thought!" [28]

AS THE POEM fragment above suggests, there are two conflicting emotions accompanying the fear of death: 1) the *desire* for immortality, and 2) the *dread* of immortality. This is the first of Kant's practical postulates. The arguments for and against these are usually couched in terms of proofs or disproofs—as are many propositions in philosophy (what some denigrate as "coercive philosophy"). There are at least two exceptions with respect to this: 1) Kant's own practical argument based on the moral necessity of an afterlife, and 2) Heidegger's notion of truth as put forth in his later work *Was Heist Denken?*—which can be translated in two different ways, both of which apply: what is called thinking and what calls for thinking. With respect to truth, he was of the opinion that Plato, and those following him, have led us astray by concentrating on "getting things right." Heidegger, on the other hand, thought that truth was mainly about "unconcealment"— that is, uncovering that which is largely concealed. It is also the primary method of getting at the heart of Being, and indeed at all three of Kant's practical postulates. (Note: This also accompanied Heidegger's turn toward poetic language and away from the stilted and formalistic language of traditional philosophy and science. He argued that the technical language of traditional investigation is ill-equipped to uncover Being.)

The idea of the "soul" is central to this discussion since it eventually leads to the idea of the "self." This is a large, complicated topic and thus can only be touched upon superficially. There is good general evidence, however, for the notion that the self involves more than just the individual. It also involves the collective unconscious of the race (see Peter Watson's ambitious, multivolume work *Ideas: A History*). Periodically and for various reasons, there is a reflective turn in attitude which Watson calls a "turning inwards" on the part of mankind—what one critic has referred to as mankind's "interiority complex." Examples include: the Axial Age (named by Karl Jaspers; from roughly the seventh to the fourth century BC when traditional religions had become mired in public ritual and prophets arose calling for personal examination and inward holiness instead); from the first to the fifth century AD (from Christ to Augustine); from the twelfth century, from the Roman Church's Fourth Lateran Council, which ordered regular confession to be made; from the fourteenth century and the Black Death in Europe; from the fifteenth century Renaissance (the rise of autobiography); from the sixteenth century, Martin Luther, and the Protestant Reformation; from the seventeenth century and Descartes; from the late eighteenth and early nineteenth centuries and Romanticism—the reaction against the Enlightenment and its attitude that reason and science could answer all questions. (According to one scholar, the essence of Romanticism and all inward turnings is the notion of Homo Duplex, a second higher self and a better one that one is trying to discover.) And finally from the twentieth century, the last great inward turning: Freud's unconscious and the attempt to be scientific about our inner life (which has been a qualified failure, according to experts).

Alcestis

This play by Euripides was presented at the annual Dionysian festival in Athens in 438 BC. It was awarded second prize. (At these festivals, each Tragedian presented a tetralogy of works . . . three tragedies and a short satyr, or seriocomic, satire play. Although there has been debate over the years about its classification, there is little doubt that it contains elements of both tragedy and comedy and is therefore probably a classified correctly as a satyr play.)

Before the start of the play, the three Fates grant King Admetus of Thessaly (the husband of Alcestis) the privilege of living past his allotted time. They were persuaded of this by Apollo, who wanted to reward Admetus for his previous gesture of hospitality. There is one condition attached to this, however: when Death comes to claim Admetus, he must have an agreeable substitute in place. The time of Admetus' death has come, and he is still without a willing replacement. His elderly parents have refused. Finally his loving wife, Alcestis, agrees to die in his place. At the start of the play, she is near death.

In the play's prologue, Apollo is seen coming from Admetus' palace, and he tells of the events leading to the present. He also hails the arrival of Death (Thanatos) who has come to lead Alcestis to the underworld. Apollo and Thanatos engage in a battle of sarcastic banter. In the end, Apollo storms out, prophesying the arrival of one (Heracles) who will steal Alcestis away from Death. Then comes the entry of the chorus who lament the situation with Alcestis. Following this, the first act (episode) begins with the entrance of a tearful maidservant. When asked for news about Alcestis, she replies, "She is alive. And dead." On her deathbed, Alcestis requests of Admetus that he not marry again, nor forget her. Admetus agrees and promises to abstain from merrymaking and generally honor her memory. Alcestis then dies.

Shortly thereafter Heracles, Admetus' old friend, arrives. He is oblivious to the sorrow that has overtaken the palace, and in the interest of kindness, the latter decides not to burden Heracles with the sad news of Alcestis' death. (By doing this, Admetus has broken his promise to Alcestis about abstaining from merrymaking.) Heracles then proceeds to get drunk. He becomes so obnoxious that one of the servants fills him in on the real story. Ashamed, he decides to confront Thanatos at the time of the funerary event scheduled for Alcestis. He does, and brings back a veiled woman whom he gives to Admetus. She appears to be Alcestis, but this isn't entirely clear. What is clear, however, is that she is temporarily mute and has the appearance of an inflatable doll—or one filled with sawdust. (She has not yet crossed over the chasm separating the living from the dead!)

It has been mentioned that some critics consider this a "problem play." Is it tragedy, comedy, or a synthesis of the two? Certainly, both elements are present. Alcestis is a tragic figure, whereas Death and Heracles are comic and base, not unlike Aristophanes in Plato's *Symposium*.

The play had numerous adaptors and revisers in the seventeenth, eighteenth, and nineteenth centuries. In particular, one controversy is especially interesting. There was a tendency to ennoble Admetus, which gave rise to a bitter controversy with the young Goethe who accused this stance of being anti-historical. He noted that the Greek love of life was the central idea of Euripides' tragedies and that Euripides' Admetus considers the life left to him "worse than death."

What then is the relevance of Euripides' Alcestis to the overall subject of this work (the exploration of death)?

1. The Truth Value of Myth

Euripedes' *Alcestis* is a myth—a sacred narrative explaining how the world and the people in it came to be as they are. The main approaches/alternatives for understanding myth are: a) to ground it in reality, b) to locate its origins in the human mind/psyche, c) to center its origins in language, and d) to look upon it as a means of understanding and even creating human experience. While each has its advocates, for our purposes the fourth approach probably comes closest.

The truth value of myth, is addressed by Jean-Francois Lyotard, one of the most central of postmodernist thinkers. He confronts this in "The Post-modern Condition: A Report on Knowledge," which has become the unofficial "bible" of postmodernism. There Lyotard talks about scientific knowledge as not being the only kind of knowledge, or of having pride of place. He recognizes a distinction between scientific discourse and narrative discourse which are "language games" in the Wittgensteinian tradition. As an example, a myth justifies itself merely in the telling. The narrator does not need to prove its truth. Scientific discourse, on the other hand, cannot legitimize itself because it is a different kind of language game since it makes denotative statements which require proof. Thus myths have their own truth value. Not all knowledge comes from science. There are different paths to knowledge and truth.

2. The Difference between the Living and Nonliving:
Difference in Kind or in Degree?

As implied before, the living are often preoccupied with death—not with analyzing it, but with facing and fearing it. Philosophers, on the other hand, embody the ideal of facing death with equanimity. Montaigne, for instance, devotes a long essay to the subject: "To philosophize is to learn to die." Cicero also: to study philosophy is "nothing else but to prepare for death." And Socrates: "The true votary of philosophy is always pursuing death and dying." The poet and prose writer, however, use the specter of death to transmit lessons to the living.

But how are the living and nonliving different? In kind or in degree? A difference in kind suggests a sharp distinction between the two. In addition, there is often a component of vitalism in the living which is totally lacking in the nonliving.

According to the position of a difference in degree, everything in the universe is alive and besouled. This is called *animism*, or *panpsychism*. In other words, the continuity of nature is uninterrupted.

Into which camp does *Alcestis* fall? This is difficult to answer because there are features of both continuity and discontinuity in this myth.

3. The Self

We commonly mean by the "self" the specific being that a person is—what distinguishes one individual from another, and that part of the individual that persists over time (referred to as personal identity). One of the self's distinctive properties is its capacity for self-consciousness. One would think, therefore, if one knew anything, it would know its own nature. Yet the self is an ongoing mystery to itself.[29] As a result, selfhood has been a recurring theme for discussion and revision throughout human history.

With respect to immortality, the question that comes up is which part of the self has the potential for temporal continuity? The self is often thought of as comprising two basic components, sometimes three: a) the reflective, introspective part, b) the physical part, and c) the relational part. (Note: those components of the self which are physically embedded cannot be eternal.) Only the reflective part of the self has the potential for immortality—more specifically that part of the "I" (the ego) which has the capacity for reflexive self-reference. When I reflexively self-refer, I known that I am referring to myself, but how do I know this? If there is an underlying, preexisting I, this gives rise to an intractable problem. For example, any being that claims to know itself through reflection must already know itself in some pre-reflective way or it could not recognize itself in the reflective mirror. In addition, introspection by itself cannot tell me that the consciousness I attribute to myself is not yours as well (a so-called misidentification error).

However, if there is no preexisting I and the I is synthesized around the act of reflexive self-reference, then there is no possibility of a misidentification error. (Still, there is no denying that there is an intuitive fitness to the view that the self exists independently.)

Thus, although some may find the above self-synthesizing view to be objectionable in that it does not locate the self as an entity, there is another way of understanding the self which explains certain persisting puzzles about the self, according to Nozick. That is, we might understand the self as a property rather than as an object. One puzzle it helps explain is Hume's famous observation about not being able to find the self. As he wrote: "For my part, when I enter most intimately into what I call myself, I always stumble on some particular perception or other. . . . I never catch myself at any time without a perception."[30] If the self were a property, this is the result we'd expect since the self could not be found as an object of introspection. As Nozick also notes, this view of the self as a property helps illuminate talk in some Eastern traditions about the self merging with the One—in other words, the self doesn't stay separate from the One, but it does not disappear either. This may satisfy some individual's desire concerning immortality. This would have additional advantages: it could potentially minimize the energy expenditure surrounding the One—that is, the total energy would remain identical (the law of conservation of "energy") for all time, in the creation and absorption of new selves; and it does not require a master intelligence, although it doesn't rule out that possibility. In other words, the universe could, or might not, be an accident of physics with biochemical trimmings thrown in.

NINE

CASE STUDIES IN PAIN

IT IS CLEAR that one mind can never know for sure what another mind is thinking or experiencing. Language and observation can give some clues, but never enough to fully reveal the private world of another. There are, of course, degrees to this *epistemologic divide*—this chasm between different minds—which narrows or widens depending upon the content being exchanged. Communicating about matter-of-fact mental images, for instance, is easier than trying to make one mind understand another's feelings or sensations. And perhaps nowhere is this gap greater than when the subject is *pain*.

In her classic treatise on the subject, Elaine Scarry makes the claim that to have pain is "to have certainty" (about one's experience of it—indeed, about one's very existence), while to hear of another's pain is "to have doubt" (about that other's experience).[31] This doubt arises because the experience is largely incommunicable. Pain, it seems, has a tendency both to *resist* language and to *destroy* it. (The phenomenon of *suffering* is similar, though not identical. Suffering can be caused by both physical and psychological pain: loss of a loved one, loss of work, betrayal, isolation, memory failure, etc. The common denominator is anything which threatens to destroy the unity of the person as a whole.)

Medicine more than any other profession deals with pain. In some sense the science of medicine is the science of pain. Yet paradoxically, its practitioners seem more opaque than most to its nonscientific dimensions. It would not be too outrageous, in fact, to accuse the profession of contributing to the *epistemologic divide* between itself and the patient in pain. Asclepius, no doubt, would agree.

Scene II

The same rocky promontory as in Scene I (chapter three). This time, however, the tree above the two stone seats is barren. Clouds again cover the sky, but they seem darker, more primordial, than before. Their density is such that even Zeus' palace (upper stage right) is almost obliterated from view. Asclepius is seated alone with his staff and is again gazing earthward in total concentration. After a few moments Hermes enters (stage right), carrying his familiar caduceus.

Hermes: Good day, Asclepius. *(He reaches his stone seat and sits next to Asclepius, but the latter seems oblivious to his entrance.)*

Asclepius: *(looking up after a few moments)* I beg your pardon, Hermes.

Hermes: You seemed distracted, my friend.

Asclepius: I was looking at something below . . . one of those shiny new hospitals with all of its gadgetry and . . .

Hermes: *(He nods, interrupting.)* Medicine certainly has progressed since our friend, Hippocrates, walked the earth.

Asclepius: The scene below did not suggest "progress" to me.

Hermes: Direct my gaze there so that I may see it too.

Asclepius: It is over now. Besides, it is something you and I have observed often enough . . . of late.

Hermes: No matter! Mankind is prone to repetition, and we will witness it again. But tell me: What was it you saw there?

Asclepius: I saw a group of physicians huddled around an old man who was near death. Against his protestations, they were busy inserting tubes and needles into every imaginable place—though he was conscious and obviously in great pain.

Hermes: They were merely trying to save his life!

Asclepius: If I had not known that the scene below was a hospital, I might have easily mistaken it for a confession chamber in one of Tiberius' palaces. *(He sighs.)* They seemed insensitive to his pain, much of which they were causing themselves.

Hermes: Of late, you seem to have grown particularly critical of your profession, Asclepius. And cynical too! That is not like you. Cynicism is my domain, not yours.

Asclepius: I suppose you are right. But it is difficult to avoid it when one sees images like that. *(He strokes the body of the serpent entwined around his staff.)* It sometimes seems that modern medicine causes more suffering and pain than it alleviates.

Hermes: I almost hesitate to ask, for surely you will blame me again for many of medicine's woes. But I will nevertheless: Why do you suppose physicians are insensitive to their patient's suffering?

Asclepius: When we were last together, we discussed the ideas of Descartes . . .

Hermes: His separation of mind from matter—the person from the body?

Asclepius: *(nodding)* Then, the commercialization of medicine . . .

Hermes: Ah! You certainly blame me squarely for that!

Asclepius: As the god of commerce, certainly you had a role in it. By treating patients as things—as commodities—you helped to transform medicine from a profession into a trade.

Hermes: So, Descartes and I are to blame for medicine's insensitivity to its patients' suffering?

Asclepius:	Only partially. *(He pauses and again strokes his serpent's brow.)* The real culprit is another.
Hermes:	At last, a temporary reprieve! But tell me, who is the guilty party? Another god? Perhaps Zeus himself?
Asclepius:	None of them, to be sure. No. The culprit is *pain* itself.
Hermes:	That sounds more like a riddle . . . or a paradox.
Asclepius:	It *is* a paradox. Pain itself drives a wedge between the sufferer and the one observing it. Perhaps a story will help illuminate this.
Hermes:	Ah . . . you remember my weakness for narratives.
Asclepius:	It is a very old one, written in an age when we still played an active role in the affairs of men.
Hermes:	You don't mean . . .
Asclepius:	Yes . . . the ancient Greeks and their great dramatists. Do you remember *Philoctetes*?
Hermes:	Only that it was written by Sophocles and the Trojan War was its background.
Asclepius:	*(He nods.)* The scene opens on the island of Lemnos, ten years after Philoctetes has been marooned there by Odysseus and the other leaders of the Greek expedition against Troy. On their way to battle, Philoctetes had been bitten on the foot by an adder, and the wound turned into a festering sore which caused him excruciating pain. Eventually, the sight and sound of his suffering became so disagreeable to his companions, they decided to cast him away on that deserted island. In the words of Odysseus himself: "We had no peace with him: at the holy festivals, we dared not touch the wine and meat; he screamed and groaned so, and those terrible cries of his brought ill luck on our celebrations; all the camp was haunted by him."
Hermes:	I remember now.

Asclepius: But they were not completely heartless in the matter, as Sophocles relates:

>He was allowed to keep the magic bow and arrows—the gift of Hercules—to hunt and to defend himself. It was indeed a godly weapon because it never missed its mark; it struck down whatever it was aimed against.

Hermes: Indeed, I recall the magic bow of Hercules. But forgive my interruption.

Asclepius: Although the Greek army had laid siege to Troy for many years, victory always eluded them. Finally, a prophet informs them that triumph can only be assured if Philoctetes—who now understandably despises the Greeks—and his magic bow are returned to the battlefield. Odysseus and Neoptolemus, the son of Achilles, are dispatched to retrieve him through guile. The young Neoptolemus is to be the innocent foil while Ulysses remains out of sight. The remainder of the play is pretty standard fare, I am afraid. Neoptolemus convinces Philoctetes to leave the island but is overcome by a sense of guilt at the last minute. Finally, the spirit of Hercules himself appears and convinces Philoctetes to leave with them. And thus Troy is finally won.

Hermes: Asclepius, you are indeed the best storyteller on all of Olympus. *(He picks up his staff from its resting place and strokes his two serpents.)* But I became so engrossed in your story that I have forgotten the question which called it forth in the first place.

Asclepius: The question, my friend, concerns the paradox of pain. Instead of eliciting sympathy, why does it so often drive a wedge between the sufferer and the observer?

Hermes: Ah, yes . . . and the answer?

Asclepius: Because pain turns one into an exile. Just as Philoctetes was marooned on his island, so those in pain are cast off on theirs.

Hermes: Why is that, do you suppose?

Asclepius: As with the Greeks and Philoctetes, it is because the spectacle is unbearable. Although there is superficial sympathy for those in pain, underneath there is also unconscious revulsion. *(He pauses.)* The only solution then is to separate oneself—geographically or psychologically—from the sufferer.

Hermes: You mean as a defense mechanism?

Asclepius: Exactly.

Hermes: And you believe that physicians are worse than others in this regard?

Asclepius: I do! Because they are constantly surrounded by those in pain, they have developed this defense better than anyone.

Hermes: *(sighing)* It is a pity that Man is such a puny animal . . . if only the gods could create him anew.

Asclepius: Yes.

Hermes: But where would our amusement come from then? Without Man we would have little to keep us so agreeably occupied.

Asclepius: Yes. We need Man more than he needs us.

Curtain

Case Studies

Following graduation, I began a residency in internal medicine—that field dealing with the immense spectrum of nonsurgical adult diseases. It was there that I first became aware of the *epistemologic divide* separating the patient in pain from his physician. Although hints of it were present everywhere in our daily routine, nowhere was it more evident than during "morning report" when patients admitted from the night before were discussed in detail. For nearly every case studied, this chasm was there for those willing to see it.

Study #1

Frank was a forty-year-old man who was hospitalized during my first month of training. He was a regular on the teaching service, and when the admitting intern presented his case at morning report, just the mention of his name caused the senior residents in the room to groan in unison like a rehearsed chorus. Frank had chronic pancreatitis—the result of heavy drinking—and every few months he would require hospitalization for his flare-ups of abdominal pain and vomiting. To complicate matters, he had also become addicted to narcotics.

"What treatment did you begin in the emergency room?" the attending physician asked the new intern after he had finished presenting Frank's case.

"I placed a nasogastric tube in his stomach to relieve the vomiting," he replied. "And I gave him intravenous fluids and pain medication."

"What kind of pain medication?"

"Morphine."

"And how did he respond to the narcotic?" He looked at the intern again.

"He only got partial relief . . . and kept asking for more."

"And you gave in to his requests . . . Frank of all people?" He smiled. "But then, how could you know." The intern looked embarrassed. "Well, I wouldn't be too upset. After all, it is part of your education to learn how some people manipulate the system to their own advantage—and pain is one of their most important tools." He paused for a moment. "How does one go about deciding how much pain someone is having?"

"I . . . I'm not sure," the intern responded.

"How do you decide?" he asked.

"Well, there are certain physiological signs that can offer clues: sweating and a change in heart rate, for example. They are not very reliable, though. I guess, in the end, it depends on your intuition. Your instinct."

"Yes. And that only comes with experience, which you should get plenty of with our patients on the teaching service. Unfortunately, you will have to match wits with experts who use pain as a weapon to get what they want—which is usually more narcotics or a hospital bed. By the way," he asked, looking at one of the residents, "how many times has Frank been admitted within the last year?"

"Eight or ten times . . . at least. The last time was two months ago. He created quite a stir, if you recall."

"Ah, I certainly do! Why don't you tell our new interns about it? It should help make my point."

"Let's see . . . we admitted Frank for his usual flare-up of pain," the resident began. "Naturally, we gave him his ration of narcotics and kept a small nasogastric tube in him to help monitor his fluid intake. For the first day he seemed to improve. But the next afternoon his pain got worse. When we evaluated him to see if any complications had developed, we couldn't find any, so we increased his narcotic dose. But the next afternoon the same thing happened . . . and then the next. In fact, the pain came on every afternoon at about the same time for nearly a week."

"Do you have any ideas about this mysterious afternoon illness?" the attending physician asked Frank's intern.

"No."

"Don't feel badly," he replied. "Neither did we."

The resident continued his story. "After this had gone on for nearly a week, we asked the nurse in charge to keep a close watch on Frank's room and to report anything unusual. After a few days, she solved the mystery for us." He grinned. "Frank, it seems, had a girlfriend who visited him every afternoon. Each time, she brought a pint of vodka with her and when the nurse left the room, she poured it down Frank's nasogastric tube." He smiled. "The nurse discovered it when she suctioned the tube and thought the contents smelled a little funny. We cured his mysterious disease simply by banning all visitors."

"You must give the man credit," the attending physician laughed. "Frank got both his alcohol and his narcotics. Very ingenious!" He looked at the intern, whose face had now taken on a burgundy hue. "Make sure you write an order that Frank is to have no visitors."

"I . . . I will," the intern said."

"No harm done. Besides, you have learned an important lesson here: be suspicious of patients when it comes to pain."

"Assume they are guilty until proven innocent?" the intern responded.

"I like that. It's a good motto," the attending physician responded. "Well then, tell us about your next admission." He sat back comfortably and stared at the wall.

Study #2

Near the end of my second year of residency, Madeline H. was admitted to the surgical service with a badly infected skin graft. As internists we were consulted to help them manage her antibiotics. She was about thirty then, and the story of her illness was especially tragic.

Ten years before, Madeline and her fiancé had been driving home from a friend's house when their car skidded off an icy stretch of highway and caught fire. He was killed immediately, and Madeline, who suffered third degree burns to much of her face and upper torso, as well as amputations of both legs (just below the knees), was hospitalized for six months. On a number of occasions, she nearly died from complications, but each time she managed to pull through. In the end, she was left crippled and, in spite of multiple surgeries and skin grafts, severely disfigured.

During her hospitalization Madeline went through the usual bouts of depression. Then toward the end of it, she suddenly—almost miraculously, one might say—came to grips with her disabilities. After being discharged she completed college and then went to work in a nursing home where her principal responsibility was to tend to the morale of the elderly residents. Never complaining about her own disfigurement and chronic pain, she seemed the closest thing to a genuine martyr that any of them had ever seen. As for Madeline, working with them gave her own life a new perspective and sense of purpose.

But when the intern and I entered her room for the first time that day, we were not prepared for the dramatic disparity between what filled our ears and what met our eyes. She greeted us cheerfully in a voice that had a lyrical lilt—almost a siren's quality—suggesting sensuous beauty. This contrasted cruelly with her tautly scarred face, which looked as if the skin there had been stretched over a network of irregular fibers laid just below the surface. The disfigurations obviously made it difficult, perhaps even painful, for her to speak or to smile.

As we examined the graft on her neck and right shoulder, she continued her buoyant conversation. It was obvious from the wound's redness and warmth that it would require aggressive antibiotic therapy and debridement. Since my intern had a full complement of patients, I decided to follow Madeline myself. After finishing the examination then, I went alone to the nursing station to review her medical records. Aside from their sheer volume, the most striking thing was that on the cover of each, stamped in bold red letters, was the instruction: *No Pain Medication of Any Kind (by Request of the Patient).* My curiosity about its significance faded, however, as I became engrossed in the medical details of her many admissions.

In the days that followed, Madeline and I gradually established a comfortable rapport. Our daily visits became something we both looked forward to. By the end of the first week, she was well enough to have the wound site prepared for another skin graft. When she had recovered from the anesthesia and was returned to the room, I came in just as the attendants were transferring her from the gurney to the bed.

"How do you feel?" I asked after the others had left. There was a bulky dressing on her neck which made her look particularly uncomfortable.

"I'm fine," she replied.

"Can I get you anything?"

"No, but thanks just the same."

"Still, it must be uncomfortable . . . now that the anesthesia has worn off." I noticed that the bulky dressing forced her head awkwardly to the right.

"It doesn't bother me . . . really."

"I'd be happy to order something for you," I insisted. Then I remembered the instructions on the cover of her medical record. "I'm sorry. I forgot that you don't take pain medications." It was the first time it had come up in our conversations.

"You find that curious, don't you?" she asked after a long pause.

"Yes, a little—considering everything you've been through."

"How much pain do you think I am having right now?"

"I'm not sure. People react so differently to it."

She nodded. "It must be nearly impossible to tell how much pain someone is in." There was a hint of sympathy in her voice.

"I'm afraid that physicians become a little hardened to patients who complain too much. I suppose, it makes us less sympathetic and . . ."

"And less likely to believe them?"

"Why, yes, but . . ."

"You forget. I am an expert when it comes to doctors and hospitals."

"Of course. Forgive me."

She looked awkward lying there on her side, and I got up to help her into a sitting position. After placing several pillows behind her lower back and shoulders, she seemed more comfortable.

"I suppose it's natural to erect a wall between yourself and your patients," she continued. "Too much emotional involvement clouds objectivity. Isn't that the argument?"

"Or perhaps our rationalization of it."

"It seems strange that I should be the one defending your profession while you find fault with it." She grimaced slightly as she turned in bed to get into a more natural position. "But there is one thing that I do criticize."

"What's that?"

"Medicine's ignorance when it comes to the matter of *suffering*," she answered soberly.

"What do you mean exactly?"

"Rather than trying to explain it, let me give you a real-life example." Her voice quivered slightly. "I had just started college when my mother was diagnosed with breast cancer. In less than a year, she was dead."

"I'm sorry."

"You needn't be. It was living that was the difficult part for her. In any case, by the time the diagnosis was made, the cancer had spread everywhere. The doctors tried to arrest it with chemotherapy and radiation, but all that did was to prolong her misery."

She tried to smile. The effort was clearly painful. I wanted to say something to comfort her, but the words would not come.

"She had persistent nausea and vomiting—and horrible pain. But worst of all, the treatments destroyed her ability to work." Madeline sighed. "You see, my mother was an accomplished painter. The treatments affected her finger movements so that she couldn't even hold a brush in her hand." She glanced away to conceal her reawakened grief. "In a way, her painting *was* her identity. When I went off to college, it became the one thing that gave her existence a sense of meaning." She looked at me and again tried to smile. "And that is what I mean by suffering: the slow destruction of one's identity—and being aware of it while it is happening."

"It sounds as if her doctors caused more suffering than the cancer did!"

"Worse yet, they seemed ignorant of it. I don't think one of them ever sat down with my mother to talk about the things that were important in her life—painting, for instance—and how the treatments might affect them." There was a pause. "There is one consolation, however," she said in a whisper. "At least she didn't live long enough to witness my own condition."

Just then the door opened and a half dozen surgical residents and medical students filed in. I got up and stepped out of the way as they surrounded her bedside. Two of them began removing the dressings, while the nurse brought a wrapped packet of sterile debridement instruments. I knew it would take them some time to finish their work, so I slipped out quietly.

The next morning I visited Madeline after rounding on my other patients. She was out of bed and sitting in her wheelchair. As I entered, she looked up at me with that pained smile which had become so familiar.

"You disappeared without saying good-bye," she scolded.

"I knew your surgeons would require time, and I didn't want to get in their way."

"In a few more days they're going to try another skin graft," she said.

"That is good news." I moved the chair close to her. "But I am still curious about that note in your chart. With the surgeons interrupting us, you never got around to . . ."

"You mean, why I refuse to take pain medication?" She looked confined and uneasy sitting there in the wheelchair.

"Can I get you some water or a soda?" I asked, looking around her room and wondering how anyone could heal in such a sterile environment. The only things that added a human touch were two framed photographs of her mother and fiancé resting prominently on the small bedside table.

"Some soda would be nice. On second thought, why don't you push me down the hall to the waiting room. It has a vending machine, and I doubt that anyone will be there yet. Best of all, it's bright and warm."

I wheeled Madeline the short distance to the waiting room. It was empty, and the cordial sunlight reached out everywhere, making it infinitely more cheerful than her own dark room. I got two sodas from the machine, then sat opposite her by the windows.

"Before I explain that note," she began, "I need to tell you something about my first hospitalization. For two or three months after the accident, no one knew for sure whether I would live or die. I had one operation after another, and each was followed by some kind of complication. At that point, I welcomed the numbing medications they gave me. Then after a few more months, I turned the corner." She stopped for a moment to take a sip of her drink. "It was then—knowing I would survive—that it suddenly occurred to me what my future would be like: crippled and hideous looking and, perhaps worst of all, in constant pain. Needless to say, I became very depressed. Then one day, when the pain was particularly severe, the nurse didn't show up with my medication as usual. I rang for what seemed an eternity and still no one came. Finally, I gave up; it was then . . ."

At that moment a young couple came in and sat down in the far corner of the room. They looked very somber, and it was apparent that they did not want company any more than we did.

"Let me take you back to your room," I said. "We can finish talking there."

As I wheeled her back down the hall to her small compartment, the sterile atmosphere again engulfed us. It seemed to tire Madeline. I called the nurse to help me put her into bed. After she left, I moved the chair close to her.

"What happened then?" I asked.

"Well, I became very frightened when I couldn't get the nurse. I thought: What if the pain becomes so terrible that I can't stand it? Suddenly my whole body began to feel very heavy. And as the sensation became more intense, it seemed as if I had become the densest object in the entire universe." There was a brief pause. "Everything else around me was so light and airy that it literally evaporated. It was as if the pain had annihilated the whole external world . . . leaving me as its only object."[32]

Drops of warm sweat had started to coalesce on Madeline's face. I got up, soaked a washcloth in cold water, and placed it on her forehead. She held it there for nearly a minute.

"I can come back later after you have rested."

She shook her head. "I've gone too far not to finish it now." She took a deep breath. "It was at that moment—when everything around me seemed to evaporate—that I felt a profound sense of peace. This may sound crazy, but it seemed as if a new world had miraculously floated in to fill the vacuum left by the disappearance of the old one." Madeline paused. "Suddenly my pain and my disabilities didn't matter any longer."

"You mean that the pain made this possible?"

"Yes. It opened a door on something that was . . . well, almost religious." She hesitated. "Please don't take what I am going to say as arrogance, but I believe the early martyrs may have experienced something similar. Some of them probably reached a point during torture where the pain became so severe—and their attention so focused on themselves—that the external world literally disappeared, allowing another to take its place."

"I don't know what to say."

Madeline sighed. "Perhaps someday you will be able to explain it all away as some strange distortion in brain chemistry. But for me, the encounter was as real as this bed I'm lying on."

"And so you've sworn off all pain medication . . . and you tolerate the discomfort as a reminder of that other world?"

"Something like that. Although I have only had the experience a few times, the presence of pain seems to keep me on the verge of it."

I looked closely at Madeline. It was as if I were really seeing her for the first time. No amount of disfigurement could mask the radiance that stared out at me. Like her "other world," there was another reality there that seemed poised to vanquish the distortions of mere appearance.

Madeline remained in the hospital for another week, and although I visited her daily, the subject of pain never came up again. After that, I didn't see her for another six months—until she was admitted for the last time. The story of her final illness was sketchy, but from its fragments and my own personal knowledge of her, I was able to piece together a logical sequence of events.

Madeline had returned to work at the nursing home after her hospitalization. Then, several weeks later, she began experiencing symptoms of depression, which became troublesome enough for her to consult a psychiatrist. It is unclear why she had suddenly become depressed, but the psychiatrist apparently thought it serious enough to prescribe an antidepressant. I'm certain that she mentioned her aversion to analgesics while he, in turn, probably assured her there was no cross-reactivity between the two groups of medications (although antidepressants are commonly used in conjunction with analgesics to alleviate certain painful conditions). Knowing Madeline as I did, it is improbable that she would have agreed to take the medication had she been aware of that.

What happened next is only speculation, but the hypothesis that emerges is a coherent one. After about a month or so of taking the antidepressant, her pain probably diminished. At the same time, it paradoxically worsened her depression—because the thing she found "sacred" (her pain) had been taken from her. The dose of antidepressant was then increased, causing a vicious spiral, and at some point her condition became hopeless to her. Knowing Madeline as I did, the method she chose to end her suffering was appropriate: drinking concentrated lye—an agonizingly slow process—possibly in an attempt to experience that more perfect world one final time.

Madeline was barely conscious when the ambulance brought her in that day. By the following morning, when the surgeons informed me of her admission, she had slipped into a coma. Until the end I visited her several times a day, as did one co-worker from the nursing home. The only other person who took a special interest in Madeline was an older nurse who had taken care of her after the original accident.

"She has been through so much," she remarked to me on that final day.

"Yes . . ." I agreed solemnly.

"Her life couldn't have been very pleasant," she said, sighing. "But I can't understand why anyone would choose such a horrible way to end it all!"

"I can't either," I lied.

"Still, the coma is a blessing." She took her eyes off Madeline for a moment and looked at me. "She doesn't feel anything now, does she?"

"No." Yet, in spite of my medical knowledge, I was not entirely convinced. Madeline looked very peaceful just then—as I imagined a martyr glimpsing a better world might look.

Study #3

Toward the end of my training, a curious patient was transferred to our facility from a small, rural hospital a hundred miles away. Mr. N. was about thirty years old and had undergone emergency surgery for suspected bowel obstruction. Although none was identified, the procedure was complicated by severe hemorrhaging due to the accidental laceration of a blood vessel by the surgeon. As a result, the patient went into shock, and although he was successfully resuscitated, his kidneys were damaged in the process. Since that hospital had no facilities for dialysis, I was contacted about transferring the patient to our facility. (As the chief resident, I was responsible for approving such requests.) The physician who called was very relieved when I agreed to accept the transfer.

"I can't tell you how much I appreciate it," he gushed over the phone. "This man really belongs at a hospital like yours—we just don't have the facilities here to deal with acute renal failure."

"You'll send all his records and reports?"

"They are being copied now, and we'll put them in the ambulance with the patient." There was silence on the line for a moment. "But I should tell you a few things about Mr. N. that are difficult to describe in a written record."

"Go on."

"His initial presentation was . . . very dramatic to say the least. When he showed up in our emergency room, he got into a scuffle with the security guard. Then he burst into the treatment area and proceeded to vomit up blood on several nurses who were trying to stop him."

"Blood?"

"Yes. We never did figure that out. Probably a small ulcer or gastritis, but that soon stopped. In any case, we were more concerned about the possibility of an intestinal obstruction."

"Why did you suspect that?"

"For one thing, he had a history of three abdominal surgeries—the first for a gunshot wound, another for an ulcer, and the last one for an abscess. We suspected that he might have adhesions from one of these. On top of that, the X-rays looked suspicious."

"But you didn't find anything when you operated?"

"Except for a few adhesions . . . nothing at all."

"Were you able to get any records from the hospitals where he was operated on?"

"That's another strange thing. He was operated on at three different veterans' hospitals, each one in a different part of the country. When we tried to get information from them, they told us that they had no record of anybody by that name."

"What did he say about that?"

"The answer he gave seemed a little farfetched . . . but, I suppose, plausible. He told us that the care he had received at the veterans' hospitals was substandard and he decided to have his name legally changed. In that way, there would be no record of him as a veteran, and no one would be able to transfer him to one of those facilities again." There was a pause. "And when we pressed him for his real name, he threatened to sign out and go somewhere else."

"It sounds like we're going to have our hands full. Is there anything else?"

"Only that he told some pretty fantastic stories about himself. The man's either the best liar in the world or a real-life James Bond character."

"Give me a quick example," I said, not wanting to stretch out the conversation much longer.

"He told the staff he had been an intelligence officer—a captain, I believe—in Vietnam. And while he was there, he had been sent on a secret mission to kidnap an enemy general. According to him, the plan backfired and he was captured instead. Then, after being held for a month, he escaped into the jungle. He was shot during the escape (that was one of his three abdominal surgeries) and then was picked up by an American patrol a few days later."

"That is pretty wild," I admitted. "But who knows?"

"Anyway, thanks again for letting me transfer Mr. N. Let me know how he does."

"I will," I said and hung up.

Several hours later Mr. N. arrived by ambulance, stuporous and nearly in shock. Our medical team worked aggressively to restore his vital signs while the surgeons inserted a dialysis shunt in his left forearm. Later that evening he had his first treatment on the kidney machine. Over the next twelve hours, his blood pressure returned to normal, and he awoke from his uremic stupor.

It is difficult to describe the sensation I experienced upon first seeing Mr. N. It was a feeling that only intensified as his hospitalization proceeded. The word that probably comes closest is "revulsion"—although even that does not capture it. In Edgar Alan Poe's story, *The Tell-Tale Heart*, the main character murders an old man because of a not dissimilar—though purely pathological—revulsion. The motive is the victim's eye, which he finds so loathsome that it drives him to blot out its offensiveness permanently:

One of his eyes resembled that of a vulture—a pale blue eye with a film over it. Whenever it fell upon me, my blood ran cold; and so by degrees—very gradually—I made up my mind to take the life of the old man, and thus rid myself of the eye forever.

In Mr. N.'s case it was not his eye, but a curious sinister smile that I found unnervingly revolting. It was intensified by the vague notion that I had seen that same smile somewhere before.

The transferring physician had not exaggerated when he described Mr. N.'s propensity for telling outrageous stories about himself. Once he had regained consciousness, he began by telling the staff that he had completed two years of law school. Since he wasn't certain whether he really wanted to be a lawyer, he had decided to take a year off and travel in order to help him resolve his confusion. He said that his "wealthy parents" did not know where he was—nor did he want them to know until he had come to some decision about his future. He admitted that the name he had given was a fictitious one and, being familiar with the law, he was also aware of the medical profession's obligation to confidentiality. Nevertheless, he was "taking no chances." When I went in to reexamine him after he had regained consciousness, I was familiar with this evolving autobiography.

"I want to thank you . . . *from the bottom of my heart,*" he said to me as I entered his room. Each word reverberated with thick disingenuousness.

"Why?"

"For saving my life, of course."

"I didn't save your life," I replied with poorly disguised annoyance. "You have the other residents to thank for that."

"But aren't you their supervisor? And don't they work under your direction?"

"Yes."

"Why be so modest then? After all, their actions are merely an extension of your own."

The tone of his comments was annoying enough, but when I glanced at him and saw that he was smiling at me, it felt like the sound of fingernails scraping a chalkboard. Something about it was particularly sinister: the two corners of his lips appeared to move in opposite directions—one side elevated, the other depressed—and for an instant, I almost imagined that it had assumed the form of an elongated swastika. It also seemed nebulously (and painfully) familiar. As if trying to avoid a sudden bright light, I looked away.

I began examining him while consciously directing my gaze away from his face and toward the two areas I knew would be remarkable. The first was his left forearm where the shunt had been inserted. The blood-filled tubing there was secured by thick bandages, with a large loop of it still exposed and loosely taped to the skin. The second was his scarred abdomen which looked like a gridiron from the pattern of its lines. As he began relating the story of each set of scars, it became apparent that Mr. N. was well-versed in medical terminology.

"You seem to know a lot about medicine," I said.

"When you have been through as much as I have, it pays to learn as much as possible about your own diseases. And," he added arrogantly, "about the profession you have entrusted your life to."

"What do you know about this tube?" I pointed to the shunt in his left forearm.

"I know that it's used to connect me to the kidney machine."

"There is one thing I should tell you about it," I said ominously and with a sense of perverse enjoyment.

"What's that?" There was concern in his voice for the first time.

"We'll have to keep a *very* close eye on this." I taped the dressing down over his shunt snugly. "It's like having an artery exposed to the outside world—if it is cut or pulled loose, you could exsanguinate in just a few minutes." I paused dramatically. "Should that happen, put steady pressure on it *immediately* and ring for the nurse."

There was no sign of a smile on his face now. For the briefest instant my imagination concocted a sadistic scene: I saw him asleep in his room with a dark figure standing over him; suddenly, there was the flash of a surgical scalpel followed by pulsing jets of blood landing on the sheets and floor. The sound of Mr. N.'s voice brought me back to reality.

"You can be sure that I'll be very careful," he exclaimed.

"I must leave now and see my other patients," I replied and then walked out of his room.

The next day during teaching rounds, Mr. N.'s case was discussed in detail for the first time. After his history was presented by the intern, the attending physician suggested the diagnosis of Munchausen's Syndrome, a disorder named after an actual eighteenth-century German soldier, Baron von Munchausen, who was notorious for telling outlandish stories. Munchausen patients described their illnesses—which were usually feigned—in dramatically exaggerated terms. In addition, they were hospitalized frequently, showed familiarity with medical terminology, became aggressive toward others when their truthfulness was challenged, and frequently left against medical advice when their demands were not met. According to psychiatrists, most of these patients had been neglected as children and it was thought that hospitalization allowed them to compensate for this by becoming the center of attention.

Mr. N. was a perfect Munchausen candidate. Although he now had a genuine illness, it was likely that he had feigned the initial condition that had led to it. And like the real Baron, he was certainly an inventor of tall tales. Finally, several days later his aggressiveness was unmasked when a psychiatrist was called in to evaluate him. Shortly after that I was paged by the nurse to come to Mr. N.'s room.

He was sitting nervously in the chair facing the doorway with a wild look in his eyes when I entered. After seeing me standing there, that hideous smile again appeared on his lips.

"Did you ask that psychiatrist to see me?" he demanded.

"It's routine," I lied. "We ask a psychiatrist see all of our new dialysis patients."

"I don't believe you," he blurted out. "You medical people are all alike! When you don't understand something, you bring in one of those fake doctors to explain it away as some kind of mental disorder."

"You don't seem to . . ."

"There is nothing wrong with my mind," he erupted. "Certainly nothing to explain this!" He held up his left arm with its bandaged shunt. "You also know that I'm a law student . . . so I know all about malpractice." His mouth twisted again into that odious smile. "The surgeons at the other hospital certainly bungled my case—they caused my kidney failure. That's malpractice in anybody's book." He stared and then pointed at me. "And you people are just adding to my mental suffering."

"I'm sorry you feel that way," I said, trying to conceal my intense dislike for him. "But as I told you, all of our dialysis patients receive a psychiatric consultation."

Without warning, his tone suddenly changed. He became conciliatory and obsequious. "I'm sorry I got so upset," he apologized.

"I understand."

"I certainly wouldn't sue you—or your hospital," he said calmly. "All I ask is that you keep those psychiatrists away from me. They need to spend their time with patients who need their help. Besides, I know you wouldn't do anything that might force me to go somewhere else for my treatment."

"Certainly not."

"By the way," he said, "the pain in my stomach isn't relieved at all by that medicine your intern ordered for me."

"I'll change it to something stronger." I left the room without looking back.

Over the next week Mr. N. became more and more demanding of the staff. Most of it centered around pain medication, and it soon became apparent that he was an addict in addition to his other problems. After discussing the situation with the attending physician, we decided to "detoxify" him by gradually reducing his narcotics and adding a mild tranquilizer in case of withdrawal symptoms. Later that day, as I was about to leave the hospital, the intern assigned to Mr. N. paged me.

"He's become very disruptive," he exclaimed over the phone. "He seems to know that we have cut back on his narcotics.

"What has he been doing?"

"Pacing the halls . . . even going into other patients' rooms. He's telling them that we are trying to kill him."

"Did you call the security guard?"

"Yes. Mr. N.'s back in his room now, but he's still carrying on." There was a pause. "Should we increase his narcotics to quiet him down?"

"I'd rather give him more tranquilizer," I replied.

That evening from home, I checked in with the intern and resident who were on call. They reported that Mr. N. had settled down considerably and was resting in bed. Just before midnight, I called one final time.

"How is he?" I asked.

"Unfortunately, he has gotten agitated again."

In the background I could hear hurried voices and then what sounded like a heavy object striking the floor. "What was that?"

"As you can tell, I am on the phone in Mr. N.'s room. The security guard had to subdue him and knocked over a metal basin in the process."

"Why don't you increase his narcotics dose . . . a little," I replied. "And add an antipsychotic to the regimen."

"I'd also like to get some leather restraints. Even the security guard is having a hard time keeping him under control," the resident replied.

"That's fine—as long as someone stays in the room with him."

"I'll have the guard stay with him," he responded and then hung up.

Early the next morning my pager went off just as I was pulling into the hospital parking lot. It was from the nursing station on the tenth floor where most of our teaching patients were located, and as I got off the elevator there, I could see a huddle of white uniforms at the far end of the hall. They were in front of Mr. N.'s door, and when I reached the room, I saw that he was lying face up on his bed with the restraints still attached to his wrists and ankles. His skin was steel gray, and his eyes were opened widely in that familiar posture of death. The left side of the bed was soaked in blood, and the floor below it splattered with large crimson clots.

"What happened?" I asked.

"When the guard left the room to go to the bathroom, the shunt must have gotten tangled up in the restraints and pulled out," the resident responded. "When we got here, it was too late. We tried to resuscitate him, but . . ."

I moved closer to get a better look at the body. I gazed at his face for a moment. His mouth was partially open, but there was no evidence on his lips of that twisted smile. Like the blue vulture eye of Poe's character, its hideousness had been permanently erased.

"There is nothing more we can do here," I said. "We'll discuss it at morning report."

Yogi's Story

Although Mr. N.'s bizarre death had been unpredictable, I still felt a large measure of responsibility for it. Why, for instance, hadn't I just given him his usual dose of narcotics and been done with it? And why had I agreed to use physical restraints? Worse yet, why could I feel no sympathy for him either in life or in death? It was apparent, however, that the *epistemelogic divide* that I had observed in other physicians had come full circle. I was as guilty as they—perhaps more so, because I had recognized these traits in others while denying them in myself. I felt an urgent need to get away and let these things sort themselves out. (My psychiatrist friend agreed.) Several years before, I had been on a camping trip in the nearby mountains. Now with spring beginning and activities at the hospital slowing, it seemed an ideal time. So, after making arrangements for call coverage with one of the other residents,

I packed the car and left early one morning. It was a week to the day since Mr. N.'s death.

I decided on driving the back roads to take in the scenery and avoid traffic as much as possible. Although it was several hours longer that way, I knew that there would still be plenty of time to reach the campsite before dark. In spite of this effort at diversion, however, the image of Mr. N. smiling up at me from a pool of blood periodically intruded itself. And for some reason, the further away from the hospital I got, the more frequent the interruptions became.

At about noon I reached the departure point at the base of the mountain. Several hours later, after an effortless climb along clearly marked trails, I arrived at the campsite near the summit. I had met no one along the way; even better, the disturbing images of Mr. N. had abated. The campsite was located in a small, circular clearing with a stone-lined fire-pit near its center. After unpacking and setting up my tent, I foraged for some wood and returned an hour later with a three-day supply. Then I lay down to take a brief nap. It was nearly dark when I awoke.

As I was about the leave the tent to start the fire, I caught sight of something in the twilight crouching near the pile of wood. My first impression was that it was a raccoon; instead, it turned out to be a small dog. When I got close to him, he rolled over on his back and then, in a gesture of friendship, licked my hand. I noticed that he had a loose leather collar, but no metal tag with any identification. Either he had been set free by someone who wanted to get rid of him or separated from his owner on a hike through these woods. The dog did not appear emaciated, but when I opened a large tin of canned meat and offered the contents to him, he ate it quickly.

"Do you have a name?" I asked, after he had finished and was stretched out in front of me at the entrance of the tent. "Since I don't know your real one, I'll just call you 'Boy.'" I repeated the name, as if there were something familiar in the sound. That night he curled up and slept beside me in the tent.

The next morning we arose early and spent the day together hiking along the side of the mountain. He seemed anxious about keeping me in sight and followed me everywhere I went. We found a family of turtles and a few young water snakes sunning themselves on the rocks of a nearby stream, but nothing more exotic. By the time we returned to the campsite, it was near dusk. I built a fire and cooked something for both of us. Afterward we sat together at the mouth of the tent gazing into the glowing firelight.

The sight of the flames against the forest background had a mesmerizing effect. The fire seemed to phosphoresce. My eyes became heavy. Although they remained open, I felt myself drifting into that twilight between waking and dreaming. I could sense my subconscious relaxing its hold and spreading its contents like a thin veil over the yellow light. In its luminous glow I could see a circular clearing much like the one I was sitting in, only larger and ringed on its periphery by a dozen or more tents:

There were boys in shorts and sneakers going in and out of the tents, while others huddled in small groups here and there. I recognized about half of these as grade school friends. As if magically transported back to that time and place, I even saw myself sitting at the entrance to one of the tents. Gradually the setting and the individuals became more familiar. The others were from the nearby city. And two of them I recognized immediately.

One was named Lance—an obnoxious twelve-year-old who was disliked by everyone—even the other boys from the city. As a symbol of this, he was the only one to have a tent all to himself. In the unfolding glow of the fire's light, I could see him sitting alone there on its stoop, sneering as he watched the others play. The sight of him reawakened a sense of revulsion.

The other was a sixteen-year-old whom I remembered only by his nickname: Yogi. He had strangely slanted eyes, an awkward gait, and mild mental retardation—in retrospect, all signs of Down syndrome. His younger brother was there also, partly to have fun and partly to look after the older boy. With the exception of Lance, everyone was drawn to Yogi as if the sight of his abnormality awakened some basic fraternal instinct in us.

As the memories flooded back, I remembered that Yogi possessed one other quality which made him indispensable to us in that summer of long ago. Like his namesake, he was a catcher—not very good, but certainly better than any of the rest of us. And although our parents had sent us to summer camp to be close to nature, we still managed to play ball nearly every day on the makeshift field in the hollow below our site. We usually assembled there late in the afternoon and played until we were called to the mess hall for dinner. There were just enough of us to field two complete teams—with Yogi catching for both. The one exception was Lance, whom no one wanted on their team. Only Yogi, who seemed incapable of dislike for anyone, treated him with any compassion at all.

By the end of the first two weeks, we had become acclimated to the routine of camp life. A few days later, however, this was disrupted by the sudden disappearance of Yogi and his brother. The camp counselor told us they had been called home and it wasn't certain when, or if, they would return. Although we missed both brothers, it was Yogi's absence that was felt most acutely because it left us without a catcher. It was then, with uncharacteristic humility, that Lance offered to take Yogi's place. The two teams huddled to discuss the matter, and in the end we agreed to let him catch—since we wanted our games to continue.

To no one's surprise, Lance proved to be a horrible catcher. Yet in spite of that, he became almost civil for a while—being included as a part of our small adolescent society, I suppose, humanized him. But the transformation was short-lived, for when Yogi and his brother returned to camp after a five-day absence, he was cast aside without a second thought. And when the game resumed the following day, he was once more on the sidelines looking at all of us with his familiar sneer.

But even with Yogi's return, things were not the same as before. In addition to his brother, he now had another companion: a homely little dog—a birthday present from his parents. That had been the reason for their mysterious absence: his parents had come to get them for a surprise party. When Yogi was presented with his new dog, however, he lost all interest in camp. Only by agreeing to let the dog accompany him were they were able to convince him to return.

"Is . . . is . . . isn't she nice? Good girl," he said as we gathered around him to look at his new pet.

"I think she's a boy," someone remarked after seeing the dog roll onto its back.

"What's his name?" another asked.

"I . . . I . . . don't have a name," Yogi replied.

"But you oughta have a name."

"You . . . you help me then," he stuttered. "A ni . . . nice girl's name."

"How's Jane?" one of the boys asked.

"I like Linda—that's my sister's name."

Yogi stared at his homely pet for a moment. Finally he said, "I . . . I'll just call her 'Girl.'"

The two of them were inseparable, and although we resumed our games with Yogi as catcher, the dog constantly interrupted our play by getting between him and the batter. In the end it took nearly twice as long to play our game. But we tolerated it for Yogi's sake.

On a Friday afternoon, a week after Yogi's return, we played our last game of the camp season. Lance had been noticeably absent from his usual place on the sidelines when we started, although midway through we saw him watching from the small incline behind home plate. Then he disappeared again. When the game was over, the rest of us walked up the hill to the campsite while Yogi and Girl remained behind to play. Ten minutes later, as we were assembling for supper, a sudden blast—like a gun discharging—erupted from the hollow below. This was rapidly followed by a short scream, then by a hoarse cry. The camp counselor was the first one down the hill. We ran after him and, although he tried to hold us back, we arrived there simultaneously. What we saw, however, arrested our motion on the spot.

Yogi was standing near the pitcher's mound covered in blood. His arms were cradled across his deformed chest. He sobbed intermittently and with each exhalation gripped his chest more tightly. As we stared at him, it became apparent that he was grasping . . . not his own chest . . . but the bloody remains of his dog.

"May I see your dog, Yogi?" the counselor asked gently.

"No . . . No! I . . . I . . . don't want nobody to touch her," he sobbed.

"All right—but maybe we can help Girl." The counselor turned to the two boys nearest him and directed them to fetch towels and a first-aid kit from his tent.

"Can . . . can you help her?" Yogi stuttered. There was a flicker of hope in his voice.

"I don't know for sure," he said soothingly. "But we can try."

A few minutes later the two boys reappeared with the supplies. The counselor spread the towels out on the ground, opened the first-aid box, and removed some bandages and a pair of scissors. Then he helped Yogi lower his dog onto the makeshift operating field.

This was our first full view of Girl, and it was a sight we were not prepared for. Her entire right flank had been torn away, including the leg and tail which were completely missing. (When the field was searched later, all that was found were some small bone and flesh fragments, but nothing resembling an extremity.) The abdomen had also burst open and its intestines extruded. The counselor immediately placed a towel over the dog and looked at Yogi.

"How did this happen?" he asked in a calm, but firm, tone.

"She . . . she's dead?" Yogi was no longer sobbing.

The counselor nodded as he turned Yogi away from the sight. "Can you tell me what happened?"

"La . . . Lance . . ."

"Lance?" the counselor interrupted.

"I . . . I told him that Girl had some worms and . . . and that she needed to see the animal doctor wh . . . when she got home." Yogi turned to look back, but the counselor skillfully guided him farther from the scene while the rest of us moved into the breach.

"Then what did Lance do?"

"He . . . he told me that Girl didn't need no animal doctor . . . that he could help her." He turned again to look in the direction of the dog, but the wall of boys blocked his view completely.

"And then?"

"La . . . Lance said he had some medicine th . . . that would get rid of the worms. He . . . he asked me to hold her while . . ." Yogi stopped abruptly. He looked at the rest of us, and then whispered into the counselor's ear so that no one else could hear.

"What happened next?" There was unmistakable anger in the counselor's voice.

"He . . . he lit a match and touched it to the medicine. Th . . . then he threw a stick . . ."

He nodded. "You don't have to tell me anymore."

We escorted Yogi back to the campsite while the counselor remained behind to clean up. The next morning, the brothers' parents arrived to take them home. Girl's body was also taken so that they could have a formal burial service for Yogi's benefit.

Lance's parents were also contacted, but before they arrived the counselor managed to get his explanation of the incident. According to the story, Lance had brought several "cherry" bombs with him to camp, which he planned to use to frighten anyone who might torment him. In the meanwhile, he had also become envious of Yogi and the attention lavished on him by the other boys. In any case, after the final game he found himself alone on the field with Yogi and Girl. When Yogi mentioned that the dog had worms, the idea occurred to Lance to insert the powerful explosive into its rectum. He "didn't know" that it would kill the dog. But other than that recognition, he displayed little remorse for the pain inflicted upon the animal—or upon Yogi.

When his parents arrived, the whole camp turned out with an avenging sense of curiosity. Through the flickering fire, I saw myself standing close to his tent as he walked out. Instead of continuing, however, Lance stopped directly in front of me and then stared into my eyes. Gradually, a hideous smile began to distort his mouth which assumed the shape of a twisted cross. I tried to glance away, but something held me to the spot. I could neither turn away from the loathsome image nor close my eyes to it.

Suddenly, I felt an attack of nausea coming on. Not the run-of-the-mill medical variety, but the kind that Sartre described as a prelude to genuine, existential *Angst*:

. . . the nausea is *inside* me; I feel it *out there*, in the wall . . . everywhere around me . . . *I am the one who is within it.*

TEN

THE JOURNAL

METAPHORICALLY, LIFE IS like a cone. When younger, our focus is on the broad end and its seemingly unlimited possibilities; when older, the concentration is more on the point where the lines converge. It's not that growing older limits the enthusiasm surrounding such opportunity, but it does imply that there are fewer roads to travel and that each must be chosen with care . . . lest true existential guilt follow in its wake. That is, every choice means the death of all other related possibilities—which is the equivalent of creating pockets of "nothingness" in our world. So we must choose our activities carefully in order to minimize any sense of existential guilt.

Although some consider "nothingness" the equivalent of death—the annihilation of being—I am beginning to think of it more as the nihilation of being (but more of that after the experiment has been completed).

The answers—if there are any—to the above may lie in the discovery of the hidden valley and a descent into the underworld (see chapter five). It's a notion that has been talked about since the ancients originated the concept and included it in their mythologies. Shakespeare may have been mistaken in this regard: death may not be "that undiscovered country from whose bourn no traveler returns." It may be the beginning of discovery.

The camp is situated in a small pocket along the extreme northern arc of the valley where I grew up. A range of medium-sized mountains abuts it there, protruding over the valley's rim like church towers above the roof-line of a medieval village. By the middle of August, when the counselors and campers have all gone home for the summer, it's deserted except for a solitary caretaker—an old man who patrols the central section once a day in his ancient truck. This is but a small fraction of its total area, however, and the rest is accessible only by scattered trails which, in late summer, are still heavily overgrown. It is to these wilderness areas—where the obscure valley, described long ago around a campfire, is rumored to exist—that I have returned each of the last ten-plus summers to see for myself.

I began by carefully mapping the camp into four quadrants and then proceeding clockwise from east to north. Intentionally or not, this turned out to be the order of increasing difficulty of the terrain. The eastern quadrant, for instance, took two summers to complete; the southern three; and the western four. The first two are mostly flat and forested by oak and hickory, while the third is more irregular and rough, especially where it borders the fourth. It is this last quadrant which is the most difficult of all because it merges into mountainous terrain to the north.[33]

24 August 20__

I found my marker easily in the small grove of white birch: a red hand-kerchief tied at eye level around one of the trunks. It's exactly where I left it last summer and hasn't been disturbed. I've set up my base camp in the clearing adjoining it.

From the looks of it, this last quadrant will take me five or six sum-mers. It's more rugged than anything I've encountered before—in addition to being more diverse. I'm no botanist, but I can identify at least a few of the species: beech, maple, and cherry on the levels and inclines, and two or three types of hemlock and pine in the ravines. Of the smaller trees and shrubs, the only ones I can pick out with certainty are dogwood and elderberry. Farther up the slopes around the large rocks, there are several varieties of fern (although I don't know any of their names). All of this will make it nearly impossible to do anything here in a straight line. In the other quadrants I was able to hike along as if I were mowing a lawn—a linear or slightly curved path in one direction and a parallel return. But here I'll have to detour around boulders, thickets, and gullies. To make matters worse, the grade is extremely steep. Yet in spite of all of that, I shouldn't miss anything as obvious as a valley, even if it is small and disguised.

No matter how difficult the terrain, however, it will be a relief compared to this last year at the hospital. Since becoming a physician "executive," I've gained a new appreciation for the business of medicine and, most of all, the trials and tribulations of managing people—in this case, primarily physicians. But then, physicians aren't ordinary people; they're more demanding and self-centered than most. I know it's easy to be a critic, but my sense of them as primarily "tradesmen" and "technicians" has only solidified over the years. (Of course, as a member of the profession, I share in this collective guilt. But fortunately, I've been given an opportunity to try and change things for physicians-in-training at our institutions—curriculum, educational atmosphere, etc. Only time will tell whether these efforts will meet with any success.)

25 August 20__

Today I hiked to the camp's northern edge—a tiring climb of about two miles—at the end of which was a small plateau. Rising above it was the face of Quarry Mountain (clearly marked on my old map of the camp and just inside its borders). It's a very fitting name too, since this mammoth slab of rock looks as if it had been quarried out of the side of an even larger mountain. It ascends vertically for a few hundred feet, totally obscuring the view to the north, and then extends for almost a mile along an east-west axis.

The small plateau fronting it is interesting too: it appears to be a dried-up lake bed, which has been blanched by the sun to the hardness of brick. It's completely lifeless, like a petrified, geological corpse, and contrasts sharply with the dense woods surrounding it on three sides. This "strangeness" may have had something to do with what I saw while standing there and looking up toward the summit. For a split second the outline of a medieval castle materialized there; then, just as quickly, it was gone. I walked around, looking up from various angles, but it never reappeared. (I'm sure it had something to do with the direction of the late afternoon sun.)

The mirage brought to mind the King Arthur story about the Quest for the Grail, complete with its vanishing castle set amidst a Wasteland. From what I remember, several of his knights had glimpsed the castle, but because they weren't spiritually prepared, it melted away before their eyes. It took years more of wandering and initiation before it materialized again. And only then were a few of them allowed to look upon the Grail within and transform the Wasteland.

In a way, coming here summer after summer has been my own Quest. (Darryl had understood that—and, in particular, the necessity of earning one's right to the prize at the end of it all.) But what is it I'm really looking for? A physical valley? God, perhaps, or Enlightenment? And once it is found, then what? Does it all culminate in one big fizzle; or, worse yet, in the discovery that it was all a cosmic joke? Still, it seems unthinkable not to continue. On the other hand, I suppose I could wander around here for years and not discover anything at all. Most of Arthur's knights, after all, ended up that way because they hadn't made themselves worthy. (I remember Rita telling me the same thing about herself long ago.) It's probably best then to concentrate on the road, rather than what lies at the end of it.

26 August 20__

Today's trip up and back was even more tedious than yesterday's. Loose boulders were everywhere and two large ravines cut my path, forcing a lengthy detour. I didn't reach the plateau until mid-afternoon and, in order to get back before dark, I was only able to spend about an hour there. I used my time to explore along the base of the cliff: it appears to be one solid block of stone, although higher up the texture is more irregular. There are even some spots that look like recesses or caves. Unfortunately there is no way to reach that area.

The event of the day, however, was reserved for my return trip. Since it was downhill I was able to walk faster. As I was coming over a fallen tree, my right foot landed just a few feet away from a timber rattlesnake sunning itself. Fortunately, it just lay there for a moment before tightening its coil, which gave me enough time to get out of striking range. Considering I was wearing shorts and sneakers, it could have easily hit my ankle. Tomorrow I'll wear boots—and take more care around downed trees and large rocks.

27 August 20__

I tried a different approach today. Instead of cutting a new path up to the plateau, I repeated the first day's route. It got me there in less than half the time of yesterday. Then on my return, I hiked downhill through new terrain. It wasn't nearly as tiring and gave me more time to explore the face of Quarry Mountain. The more I think about it, the more certain I am that if there is an obscure valley, it must lie somewhere up there—perhaps even on the *other side* of the mountain. And if that's the case, then there might be a passageway along that wall.

I didn't find any evidence of an opening, but I did see something else interesting. While scanning the ridge, I saw a huge bird perched on a ledge below the summit. It was the same slate-gray color as the rock, which camouflaged it almost perfectly. Judging from the size, it reminded me of an eagle; but its head was black instead of white, which probably means it's a hawk of some kind. I watched for a few minutes until it glided from its perch, then soared north above the summit and finally disappeared.

I remember from somewhere that hawks were once thought to be symbols of the *divine*. Apollo's messenger was a hawk and, if I'm not mistaken, the ancient Egyptians considered it a full-blown deity. In those days it was probably easy to see gods (or God) in nature, but our world makes that extremely difficult. The main problem, I think, is a linguistic one: God is no longer a meaningful word. The only ones that seem to have meaning nowadays are those that relate to concrete things, while those that don't atrophy and become extinct.

28 August 20___

That gray hawk was back today. It was circling the plateau and seemed to follow me wherever I went. When I get home, I'll do some research and try to find out exactly what species it is. Whatever it is, there is something both magnificent and frightening about it. Rilke was right: "Beauty is nothing but the beginning of terror."

29 August 20___

The most significant thing about the geography of Quarry Mountain is that it's completely exposed for about half its length, while for the other half, its base is obscured by forest—as my crude "map" indicates:

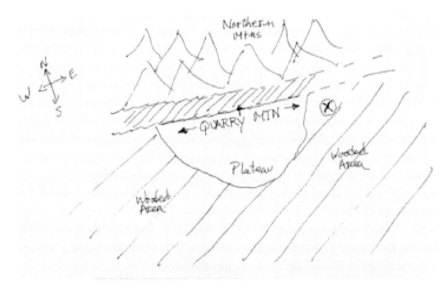

On the plateau it appears to be nothing but solid rock. But what about in that overgrown area to the east (X)? Is it densely foliated there because veins of soil extend from one side of the mountain to the other through some sort of communication (crevices, caves, etc.)?

If that turns out to be the case, then what lies on the opposite side might very well be a small valley. It would certainly fit with the counselor's story. (I can imagine the tribal elders escorting the boy up to the plateau; leading him into the woods, then through an opening into the valley on the other side; abandoning him there and waiting back on the plateau; and finally retrieving him and returning home.) Next summer then I'll set up my base camp there and begin my search in area X.

25 August 20___

I arrived on the plateau around four this afternoon. It's a perfect site for a base camp: flat, dry, and sheltered during the hottest part of the day by the shadow of the mountain. With this as my starting point, it should leave twice as much time to explore as last summer. Provided, of course, that the weather holds out . . .

. . . which doesn't look very promising right now. I shouldn't really complain though. In the ten-plus years I've been coming here, it has rained only five or six times. And those were usually quick affairs with the sky blackening suddenly and then pouring out its contents in the space of an hour. Today, however, the clouds have been accumulating more slowly, as if they had something more persistent in mind.

But there was one positive omen: that large hawk was here to greet me when I arrived. Unfortunately my research this past year came up empty. Only two looked even remotely similar: the red-shouldered and red-tailed hawks—although they're much smaller with wing spans of three to four feet, compared to five or six for this one. Perhaps it's some kind of mutation.

26 August 20___

The rain began just after dark last night and ended only a short time ago. As a result I had to spend the entire day inside. Camping here on the plateau may not have been such a good idea after all! There was a steady stream of water through the tent all day long. Luckily, I brought a cot instead of just a sleeping bag.

It did give me time, however, to finish the reading I packed in case of something like this: in addition to Rilke's poems (which I take everywhere), I brought the final volume of Tolkien's *The Lord of the Rings*. This is my fourth reading of the trilogy, and I never seem to tire of it. There's something about his style and choice of words that makes Middle Earth, Mount Doom, and their magical inhabitants almost come to life. And it seems even more so at this moment. I'm sure it has to do with this setting. Quarry Mountain, for instance, could almost be one of his fantasy mountains. Up near the top with its cavern-like recesses, I can almost imagine his race of ancient dwarves living in its labyrinth of tunnels and guarding some "treasure" deep within.

Come to think of it, isn't the labyrinth a modern symbol for meaninglessness and despair? But it's also true that most important symbols contain something of their opposite. So where did the idea of "meaninglessness" come from in the first place? Doesn't it require that the notion of "meaning" already exists?

27 August 20___

It was clear and bright when I awoke this morning, and I spent the day trying to catch up on lost time. I started by exploring the border of X where it meets the plateau, looking for an old Indian path, or some other kind of natural entranceway there. Several spots looked promising, but after following them a short distance, they merged into the underbrush. Tomorrow I'll enter at that point on the plateau where the mountain intersects directly with the woods, and then work my way along its base in an easterly direction.

Those physical "dead ends" that I encountered today just reaffirm the idea of the labyrinth. Not only is it difficult to find one's way around inside of it, but locating its entrance may be the most daunting task of all.

28 August 20__

I began working my way east along the mountain wall today. For the first twenty yards or so the foliage was very dense, then it thinned temporarily, and I was able to get in close for a look at the base. To my surprise it was discontinuous in several places (almost as if separate boulders had been fitted together there). I could even pry a stick into some of the seams. Not big openings . . . but openings nevertheless. My biggest find, however, came a short time later.

About fifty yards in was a small clearing contiguous with the mountainside and, in the center of it, a five-foot high vertical slab of stone, bleached gray-white like the floor of the plateau. It had an eerie, almost human look about it that reminded me of a Greek statue (a woman, possibly a goddess). The torso, breasts, extremities, and neck were easy to make out, but it was the face that had the greatest detail—the mouth in particular. The corners were bent down slightly, giving it an unmistakable look of sadness.

My first thought was of Persephone (even though I can't recall having ever seen a likeness of her). It may have been the hint of melancholy that suggested it. But whatever it was, it reminded me of a story I had once read about her—and as I stood there, that memory seemed to animate the statue in my imagination:

Summer had died away, and autumn's breezes filled the void. The trees were nearly bare, giving the appearance of a graveyard of bent skeletons. The statue of Persephone began to stir. She hung her head in sadness, realizing that her time to depart was near—the wind was not the wind, after all, but the hollow cries of the dead beckoning her return.

She raised her head and looked around at the transformed beauty of the forest clearing. "How can I leave all of this behind?" she said to herself sadly. Then she sighed resolutely and walked to the mountainside where a huge crevice appeared.

The earth began to tremble and in an instant she was swallowed up and hurtled into the darkness. She seemed to fall interminably. Then, as she approached that other realm, the denseness of the waiting spirits slowed her descent, and she came to a gentle stop among them. As they crowded around, welcoming her with speechless voices, she began to remember things which her brief stay above had erased— just as her brief visit here would do for those memories. Gradually, the paradoxes of death again took on clarity and she felt at home once more.

Above, autumn turned to winter and then to the first hint of early spring; below, Persephone heard the faint commotion of the stretching roots through the breach. It was her signal to return. "How can I leave these beautiful mysteries behind?" she sighed. But on the appointed day she stood in the customary spot and said good-bye to her companions. Suddenly, the two worlds cracked open and she found herself standing again in the forest clearing. And so . . . year after year . . .[34]

I looked again at the piece of motionless sculpture. The corners of its mouth were still turned down, as I imagined hers to be on those eternally recurrent days of transition.

29 August 20__

What a shame that this was my last day! About twenty-five yards east of Persephone's statue, I discovered a small cave in the mountainside—just above ground level, about three feet across. I was hesitant at first, but when I shined my flashlight and didn't see any ominous reflections, I crawled in. About three body lengths inside, the cave expanded into a small bubble where I could kneel and turn 360 degrees. Unfortunately, though, the tunnel leading forward from the chamber narrowed again after a short distance, and I couldn't go any farther in that direction.

But this is the encouraging part: as I was moving forward, my flashlight went out for a moment, and at the same time, I detected a faint glow from somewhere in front of me. Then, when I turned it off intentionally, I saw the same afterglow. It's too bad I couldn't make any more progress in that direction. Nevertheless, it's a promising sign that a passageway to the other side might be close at hand.

I should be ecstatic about this discovery, and I was at first. But now, sitting here in my tent in the lantern light, I feel an inexplicable sense of disappointment.

30 August 20__

3:15 a.m. I had the strangest dream. Rather than waiting until morning, I'm writing it down while it's still fresh (including the dialogue, some of which I'll have to "reinvent").

The setting: a small auditorium with an elevated stage and podium at one end; facing it are a dozen rows of cushioned seats with a group of children sitting in them. Two adults are standing together near the podium. Behind them is a lowered movie screen. One of them motions for silence.

"I'm afraid Uncle Pete isn't going to make it tonight," he said into the microphone.

We all groaned (I was among them), and a few of the younger children began to sob.

"Don't forget that Uncle Pete is a very busy man—he has to drive all the way from the city. That's close to a hundred miles."

"But he promised!" one of the girls cried out. "We've been waiting for this for . . ."

Just then three people in coats entered the room, and our sadness instantly melted away. Uncle Pete smiled and walked to the stage, while his two assistants set up a movie projector in the center of the room.

"Sorry I'm late, kids," he said with his charismatic smile, "but the traffic out of the city was *very* heavy tonight."

We sat down, contented now that Uncle Pete was here in the flesh. Just as he did every afternoon on his kids' television program, he began with several funny stories. Then came the part we had been waiting for.

"And now, *The Little Rascals*," he exclaimed. We all cheered. "Yes . . . just as I do every day on my show, kids, I'm going to run one of their films. And a very special one at that! It's one I've never shown before because it was only recently discovered in someone's attic. To my knowledge, it's the only movie ever made of *The Lord of the Rings*. So here they are!"

The lights dimmed, and the screen flickered to life as the familiar theme music impregnated the room. (Dah de-dah, de-dah, dahh . . . de dah de dah de dahh).

The Gang's clubhouse comes into focus: Darla, Alfalfa, Spanky, and Buckwheat are sitting at a table in front of the room. Facing them are a dozen other nameless Rascals. An old, dusty book lies open on the table. Spanky stands up and motions for silence.

"Gang," he said, "just as the Book predicted, the Dark Force has started to move. It's only a matter of months before he prevails. And you know what that means, kids—no more candy, no more movies, no more fun!"

"Tell us again where you got that old thing," one of the boys in the front row said, pointing to the Book.

Spanky turned to Darla. "I discovered it in a dusty corner of the MGM prop room," she replied. "Between the sets of *Red Dust* and *Dinner at Eight*."

"But we've been able to trace it all the way back to the time when elves and dwarfs and other enchanted beings roamed the earth," Spanky added by way of qualification.

"Wow!" the boy who asked the question exclaimed. "And what does the Book say?"

"That the Dark Force will triumph . . . unless we can somehow return the Magic Ring to the forges of Mount Doom where the dwarves first cast it out eons ago."

"Who's got the Ring now?" someone else asked.

Darla smiled. "It came with the Book . . . I have it. All that's left now is for the Ringbearer to arrive."

"Who's that?" Buckwheat asked.

"It's the stranger who will carry the Ring to Mount Doom and throw it into the fire," Spanky answered.

"Why can't it be one of us?" Alfalfa asked, looking dejected.

"Because," Darla replied, "the Book says it's got to be an outsider—someone chosen just for this task."

"When will we meet this stranger?" Buckwheat asked.

"In a minute . . . he's out *there* right now," Spanky said, pointing beyond the movie screen. "It's time. Come, Darla."

The two of them got up and walked toward the unseen camera. When they were face-to-face with it, the screen suddenly billowed out into the auditorium. The children around me screamed and began running toward the exits. For some reason, I couldn't move. A moment later I found myself sitting there alone, with the screen still expanding around me. Soon it became as thin as a membrane, covering me completely. Then, with a loud explosion, it contracted. The next thing I knew I was standing *inside* the screen with Darla and Spanky on either side of me. They pulled the last remnants of the membrane from my clothes, and we walked together to the front of the clubhouse.

"This is our Ringbearer," Darla said, holding up my arm. But instead of cheering, everyone was somber and silent.

"It will be a dangerous journey," Spanky said to me. "You will encounter trolls and orcs and other horrible creatures on the way. But you must deliver yourself—and the Ring—to Mount Doom in exactly one month." He looked at Alfalfa, Darla, and Buckwheat. "We'll go by a separate route as decoys."

"We're all pulling for you," Darla croaked, stroking my arm.

"Here is your map." Spanky handed me an ancient piece of parchment. "And," he said solemnly, "the Ring. Protect it with your life!"

It was made of a heavy substance, more lustrous than gold, in the shape of a human skull with two small rubies for eyes, which stared out at me as if they were alive.

"One more thing," Spanky said. "Keep the Ring in your pocket or another safe place. Whatever happens, do *not* put it on your finger!" I began to ask why, but he cut me off. "Because it says so in the Book."

The next part of the adventure is vague. I remember the sky blackened by hideous flying creatures and the ground vibrating to the ominous sound of patrolling orcs and trolls. When I finally arrived at the base of Mount Doom a month later, the dream became intelligible again.

Mount Doom was Quarry Mountain—but far more sinister-looking. Scanning its dark, cloud-covered peak, I couldn't imagine how I would be able to climb its sheer wall and locate the entrance to the ancient forge of the dwarves. Suddenly I spotted a patrol of orcs approaching from beneath the plateau. In a minute they would have me hemmed in between them and the wall of rock.

At the same time, there was a loud commotion overhead and I saw a gigantic gray hawk gliding gracefully along the wall. It landed beside me. As if by instinct, I gripped the soft neck feathers and pulled myself onto its back. Then we ascended quickly out of reach of the enemy. Near the summit it alighted on a wide ledge which led into a tunnel. I dismounted and followed the hawk.

The passageway was not entirely dark, and there appeared to be a source of dim light somewhere far up ahead. As we walked on, the air became warmer, and I could hear a faint din, like the sound of a waterfall. Soon I began noticing additional side tunnels which were difficult to distinguish from the main one. The only signs indicating the correctness of our path in the labyrinth were the increasing light and noise up ahead. Finally, we came to an acute angle in the passageway and, turning the corner, found ourselves in a cathedral-like cavity deep inside the mountain.

The chamber had a warm glow and a quiet roar which originated at the end of the room opposite the entrance. Suddenly Alfalfa, Buckwheat, Spanky, and Darla appeared from the shadows. We embraced each other and then walked together toward the source of light and noise. Stopping on a broad ledge, the five of us looked down into a deep abyss terminating in an ocean of orange-red lava.

"That is the forge where the ancient race of dwarves cast the Ring," Spanky said solemnly.

"You do have it—you didn't lose it?" Darla asked.

"It's right here in my pocket."

"Excellent!" Buckwheat exclaimed.

"What is it about the Ring that makes it so necessary for us to destroy it?" I asked.

"The Book says that it's a source of extraordinary power to the wearer. That's why the Dark Force wants it," Darla replied.

"But even though he doesn't possess it, he can still tap some of its energy," Spanky added. "Only this forge—where it was originally cast—is hot enough to destroy its power for good."

"What do we do now?" I asked.

"Show us the Ring first," Alfalfa said.

I took the heavy metal object out of my pocket. As I did, I felt a sudden surge of static energy course through my bones and flesh.

"You haven't tried to put it on, have you?" Darla asked.

"No . . . I followed your instructions *exactly*."

"Good! The Book says the Ringbearer must not put it on until the time has come to throw it into the fire." Spanky looked at the others for a moment and then turned to me. "It's time," he said solemnly.

I pushed the Ring onto my finger. The tingling sensation multiplied a hundredfold.

"Now, take it off," Darla commanded.

I rotated the Ring and attempted to slide it forward. It wouldn't budge. I tried several more times, but the result was always the same. "It . . . it seems to be stuck," I said nervously.

"He *is* the true Ringbearer," Spanky whispered to the others.

Just then the hawk appeared from the shadows. It stood there regally for a moment and then lowered its head as if signaling to the others. What happened next was completely unexpected. Darla came close and kissed me on the lips. I closed my eyes, and an instant later I felt myself falling into the chasm.

"We're sorry," she said calling out to me," but it was ordained that the Ring *and* its Bearer must be sacrificed."

"There was no other way," Spanky said apologetically as his voice trailed off into a whisper, blending perfectly with the faint closing strains of the *Our Gang* theme: Dah de-dah, de-dah, dahh . . . de dah de dah de dahh.

After that, I was aware only of the roar and radiation from the approaching furnace below. As the heat became more and more intense, the pain became nearly unbearable. Only the light from the forge seemed to offer any relief. Its color, which changed from a red-orange to a silvery hue, had a comforting quality which seemed to negate the inferno's blaze. Just before striking the lava, the Ring on my finger abruptly expanded, encasing me within it. I felt the hot metal diffuse into my tissues and, as it did, I had the acute sensation that time itself was being embalmed. There was no more *now*—or *before*—or *after*; they had been abolished to make room for a single, immutable instant. I knew then that I was *dead!*

When I next opened my eyes, I found myself lying on the edge of a field. The collective glow of a billion stars illuminated the darkness of the night sky. Off to my right, in the field proper, I could see the lights and hear the noises of a carnival. I pulled myself up and walked the short distance into the anonymous crowd.

There were lighted Ferris wheels and booths with all sorts of exotic attractions. The noise was intense as the barkers extolled their wares to the multitude of smiling faces. As I wandered among them, they seemed oblivious to my presence. Occasionally, however, one of the adults looked carelessly in my direction, then turned away quickly, while giving me the courtesy of a wide berth. Only the smallest children recognized me immediately and kept me in their gaze until the elders pulled them back again and scolded away their fascination.

Soon I reached the carnival's periphery and found myself alone there. I turned for one final look, then walked past the dimly lit billboards emblazoned with the word "Deathless" into the quiet meadow beyond. Here, behind the billboards and out of range of the carnival, the view became real for the first time. The stars had a pure sparkle, and the wet grass felt substantial. Shortly I was joined by two of the Laments— Sisters of Sorrow—who looked suspiciously like my own Rachael and Rita. They pointed beyond the meadow to a dim landscape of valleys and mountains just visible in the starlight.

"We live out there," Rita said, pointing in that direction.

"Yes . . . it's a very long way," Rachael added.

As we walked together, they told me the history of their people. "Once we were a powerful race," Rita explained. "Our ancestors mined those mountains for gems of pure sorrow."

"But that was long ago," Rachael said. "Before the carnival came and pushed into our valleys."

As we walked through the landscape of Lament, they pointed out the ruined temples and statues dedicated to sadness and structures only half-completed. There was almost too much to see; from the immenseness of my own recent death, I could take in only a fraction of what they had to show me.

Finally we came to a ravine, beyond which was the mountain range I had first seen in the distance. We stopped here, and the two Laments embraced me with tears in their eyes.

"You must go on alone from here," they said and began walking back along the way they had come.

Then I began my silent ascent.

EPILOGUE

IT WAS NEARLY light outside by the time I had finished writing it all down, and rather than going back to bed, I decided to pack and get an early start for home. The drive was about twelve hours, which I thought would give me time to begin deciphering the events of the past week. But it was the dream which occupied me completely.

Parts of it were obvious, even if their meanings were not. The scene from Tolkien's *The Lord of the Rings*, for instance, clearly came from that day of the downpour when I was confined to my tent. And Uncle Pete: he *had been* a real television personality who did entertain us one evening long ago with an *Our Gang* film—although I had to admit that their appearance here injected an element of absurdity into an otherwise somber dream. Finally, that carnival scene and the two Laments were right out of Rilke's *Duino Elegies*—the Tenth, to be exact, which I've read so often that each word is chiseled into my memory.

Nothing else occurred to me for the next hour as I drove the quiet back roads toward the interstate and its direct homeward path. Just before entering the main highway, I passed a colorful billboard with pictures of happy children, and for some inexplicable reason, my mind suddenly filled with images and memories of the Major—our never-completed conversation, his special gift of books, and that final brief illness all came back to me in eerie detail. These were all dissolved, however, by the unexpected appearance of his mythological alter ego: Camus' sad yet defiant Sisyphus. I could visualize the scene almost as well as my first reading of it that weekend of the Major's death thirty years before. I saw the sinewy figure straining at his burden, his brow contorted in despair and sorrow, as he pushed his rock up the sharp incline of the mountainside; reaching and pausing at the summit in a futile search for a piece of level earth to rest his load; releasing his grip and letting it roll back onto the plain below in resignation; and finally descending and beginning all over again—now, however, with a look of contentment rather than of sorrow. The words of that familiar passage from Camus also came back to me, framing in their concise beauty both Sisyphus' and our own human dilemma:

Man stands face to face with the irrational. He feels within him the longing for happiness and reason. The absurd is born of this confrontation between the human need and the unreasonable silence of the world.

Like Sisyphus, my task had also brought me face-to-face with the absurd—and its self-contained notion of fate. (But how could it be otherwise, considering the inevitability of death—the ultimate fateful absurdity?) Yet within that limit, the borders of which my apprenticeship in death had been testing, I also sensed that my fate was my own. For the most part, I was its creator . . . my life's own novelist in that regard. That mysterious hawk, for instance, had been just an ordinary bird until my consciousness had transformed it, and that statue merely a slab of stone until my imagination thought it otherwise. I had been responsible for their coherence as elements of my own story—just as I had been for Persephone and Martin, Rachel and Rita, Madeline and Darryl, and all the others—and even for the altering moods of futility and joy in its plot. And it occurred to me that, as with the endless motion of Sisyphus, my story (and "experiment") was never really meant to be completed. For as long as there was a moment of consciousness remaining, I would be forced to go on writing my own existence.

EPIMYTHIUM

FOR THOSE HEALTHCARE providers and policy makers who read this, the following is the message to be taken away:

Society, our professions, etc. seek to "normalize" us. They categorize us, assign us a role, and impose their notion of truth on us. We must, however, refuse the role we've been given. We need to remold ourselves as a sculpture, as Plotinus taught. The only way we can do this is by becoming more "authentic" in our everyday lives—which, according to Heidegger, is a difficult undertaking and requires a "bizarre" change of attitude such as Being-towards-death. In any case, the role we've been assigned must then be denied and transcended through imagination and improvisation. Only in this way can we turn constraint into freedom.

NOTES

1. Robert Nozick, *Philosophical Explanations* (Cambridge, Mass.: Belknap Press, 1981) p.1.
2. Karl Jaspers, On My Philosophy: From Dostoyevsky to Sartre, edited by Walter Kaufman (New York: Plume, 1975).
3. Albert Camus, *The Myth of Sisyphus*, translated by Justin O'Brien (New York: Vintage International, 1991), p. 20, emphasis mine.
4. William Shakespeare, *As You Like It*. The complete passage is:

Sweet are the uses of adversity,
Which, like the toad, ugly and venomous,
Wears yet a precious jewel in his head.

5. Persephone symbolizes the seed which lies concealed and dormant in winter (death), and then reappears as new vegetation in spring (life).
6. "Politics is for the moment and equation is for eternity."
7. This, and all other passages quoted from Rilke, is from the Stephen Mitchell translation: *The Collected Poetry of Rainer Maria Rilke* (New York, Vintage International, 1989).
8. She was bitten by a snake, died, and was taken to the Underworld.
9. A literary work exploring the early life of an individual with a particular emphasis on the development of character.
10. Bunny Berigan's 1938 version of the famous Gershwin song "I Can't Get Started."
11. From "Orpheus. Eurydice. Hermes" written by Rilke in 1904.
12. Michel Foucault, *Birth of the Clinic*, translated by A.M. Sheridan Smith (New York: Vintage Books, 1994). The author attributes to the pathologist Bichat the following similar statement: "Open up a few

corpses: you will dissipate at once the darkness that observation alone could not dissipate."

13. There is something about a corpse that gives it a solidity—a unique-ness—rarely noticed in life. Perhaps it is through this perception of the other's uniqueness that one's own being is sensed in its most primordial form as both an object and a subject of personal knowledge.

14. John Paul Sartre, *Nausea*, translated by Lloyd Alexander (New York: New Directions Books, 1964).

15. From "And Death Shall Have No Dominion" in *The Collected Poems of Dylan Thomas* (1934-1952) by Dylan Thomas (New York: New Directions Books, 1971).

16. William S. Burroughs, *Naked Lunch* (New York: Grove Press, 1991), p. xxxv.

17. Fyodor Dostoevsky, *The Brothers Karamazov* (New York: Everyman's Library, 1992), p.

18. This is from Michel Foucault's classic study, *Madness and Civilization*, translated by R. Howard (New York: Vintage/Random House, 1973). It was not until a few years later that I began reading Foucault. I must assume that Darryl, although he never mentioned him by name, was familiar with his works.

19. I had read this description in Burroughs' *Naked Lunch* and person-alized it for the session that day.

20. "The Gay Science," *The Portable Nietzsche*, edited and translated by Walter Caughman (New York: The Viking Portable Library, Nietzsche Collective Works, 1976) pp. 95–96.

21. The physicist Helmholtz offered a similar three-part process in de-scribing the development of a thought or idea: Preparation, Incubation, and Illumination. Helmholtz was a physicist and his scheme was aimed at the explication of scientific ideas and theories. With metaphysical questions, however, no final illumination is possible; at best we can hope for fragmentary insight.

22. From "Sunday Morning," Wallace Stevens.

23. *The Confessions of St. Augustine*, VIII, 12; The Great Books of the Western World, vol. 8 (New York: Encyclopedia Britannica, 2nd edition, 1990), p. 77.

24. *The Portable Nietzche*, p. 96.

25. Dante's *Divine Comedy* is divided into three parts or canticles: Inferno (Hell), Purgatorio (Purgatory), and Paradiso (Paradise). Each contains thirty-three canticles, assuming that the first canticle of Hell is viewed as prologue. The translation referenced here is that of Charles Singleton (Bollinngen Series 80, Vol. 1: *Inferno*; Vol. 2: *Purgatorio*; Vol. 3: *Paradiso*. 1970, 1973, and 1975 by Princeton University Press).

26. The title of Thomas Merton's autobiography, *The Seven Storey Mountain*, is a reference to Dante's seven terraces on Mount Purgatory.

27. Leah and Rachel were the Old Testament daughters of Laban and each became in turn the wife of Jacob.

28. From Joseph Addison, English essayist and poet (1672–1719).

29. Robert Nozick, *Philosophical Explanations* (Boston: Belknap Press, an imprint of Harvard University Press, 1981), p. 27.

30. Jerrold Siegel, *The Idea of the Self: Thought and Experience in Western Europe Since the Seventeenth Century* (Cambridge University Press, 2005), p. 125.

31. Elaine Scarry, *The Body in Pain* (New York: Oxford University Press), 1985.

32. This process of pain "disintegrating perception" is discussed in Scarry's book, previously cited.

33. The journal entries here are from the last two summers only. (They represent time spent exploring the northern quadrant.)

34. From a short piece "Persephone Remembers" by Irene A. Faivre (*Parabola*, Vol. XXI, No. 2, 1996).

CPSIA information can be obtained
at www.ICGtesting.com
Printed in the USA
BVHW051328210223
658921BV00012B/1093